Health Economics: an introduction for health professionals

Health Economics: an introduction for health professionals

Ceri J. Phillips
Centre for Health Economics and Policy Studies, School of Health Science,
University of Wales Swansea, Swansea, UK

Blackwell
Publishing

Books

© 2005 C.J. Phillips
Published by Blackwell Publishing Ltd
BMJ Books is an imprint of the BMJ Publishing Group Limited, used under licence

Blackwell Publishing, Inc., 350 Main Street, Malden, Massachusetts 02148–5020, USA
Blackwell Publishing Ltd, 9600 Garsington Road, Oxford OX4 2DQ, UK
Blackwell Publishing Asia Pty Ltd, 550 Swanston Street, Carlton, Victoria 3053, Australia

First published 2005

Library of Congress Cataloging-in-Publication Data

Phillips, Ceri.
  Health economics : an introduction for health professionals / Ceri J. Phillips.
    p. ; cm.
  Includes bibliographical references and index.
  ISBN-13: 978-0-7279-1849-9 (pbk.)
  ISBN-10: 0-7279-1849-4 (pbk.)
  1. Medical economics.
  [DNLM: 1. Economics, Medical. 2. Health Care Costs. 3. Health Services Needs and
Demand. W 74.1 P559h 2005] I. Title.

RA410.P49 2005
338.4′33621–dc22

                                                            2005014986

A catalogue record for this title is available from the British Library

Set in 9.5/12pt Meridien by SPI Publisher Services, Pondicherry, India
Printed and bound in India by Replika Press PVT Ltd

Commissioning Editor: Mary Banks
Development Editor: Veronica Pock
Production Controller: Debbie Wyer

For further information on Blackwell Publishing, visit our website:
http://www.blackwellpublishing.com

The publisher's policy is to use permanent paper from mills that operate a sustainable
forestry policy, and which has been manufactured from pulp processed using acid-free
and elementary chlorine-free practices. Furthermore, the publisher ensures that the text
paper and cover board used have met acceptable environmental accreditation standards.

Contents

Acknowledgements

My thanks go to all the health care professionals – dentists, doctors, nurses, occupational therapists, pharmacists, physiotherapists, psychologists – whom I have had the privilege of meeting and working with. The studies in which I have been involved have included many anatomical points from head to toe, and have given me an insight into the beauty and complexity of the human form and its amazing capacity to recover. At the same time, I have also been forced to consider what actually is of value and should be treasured. Health is a highly precious commodity and health care makes an important contribution in its protection and improvement. I therefore wish to record my thanks to the health care professionals who have been involved in my treatment and care from the cradle thus far. They are too numerous to mention but I am deeply indebted to Dr Haydn Mayo for his interest in my work, but also his dedication as a GP when one of my children was suffering from prolonged bouts of ill health.

Colleagues at a number of institutions have provided invaluable guidance and assistance over many years. Again they are too numerous to mention, but my friends at the Pain Research Unit in Oxford warrant a special note of thanks – it was Andrew Moore and Henry McQuay who persuaded me to embark on this venture!

I would also like to express my gratitude to my colleagues at Swansea who have given me the scope to write this book and the encouragement to complete it. Again, I cannot refer to everyone but must mention Shân, Sue, Angela, Ginevra and Sally for their efforts and support. My students also deserve appreciation for acting as the guinea pigs on whom most of the ideas contained in the book have been tested.

Two people – Paul Thomas and Colin Palfrey – who have tried 'since I was a boy' to initiate me into the finer points of the English language warrant thanks for their friendship, support and encouragement over too many years to contemplate.

The assistance and support of Mary Banks and Veronica Pock, Editors at BMJ Books/Blackwells, have helped smooth the process and make the effort worthwhile.

Finally Karin, Rhian, Dan and my mother Jean have had to live with 'the book' for many months, and they have accumulated many 'brownie points', which I will endeavour to repay. I accept responsibility for any errors and failings that this book contains.

Diolch yn fawr i chi gyd.

CHAPTER 1

Introduction

As policymakers and politicians grapple with the ever-increasing problem of how health services should be provided and funded, and as commentators and media correspondents devote numerous column inches and programme minutes to highlighting the problems and inadequacies of health care systems, health care professionals are increasingly being inundated by the pressures and demands placed on them to meet a variety of targets as part of contractual obligations, to provide the same (or greater) volume of services, but with fewer resources and against the background of an increasing threat of litigation if things go wrong or if patients are not satisfied.

The aim of this chapter is to provide an insight into the subject of health economics and its derivation. The chapter initially considers some of the issues confronting health care systems at the beginning of the twenty-first century and what the discipline area of economics entails. The concepts that underpin health economics – efficiency and equity – are explored, before a more detailed explanation of health economics and its relevance to health professionals. The chapter concludes with an overview of the remainder of the book.

The issue of how health services should be provided and the extent of resources required for such provision is clearly one of the most contentious political issues of the day. It continues to exercise governments and political parties of all colours and persuasions, as they attempt to offer remedies and solutions for an increasingly complex set of problems. However, aside from the short-term political controversies, there is a more fundamental issue taxing the minds of all governments in the developed world – that of what has been termed the health service dilemma.[1–3] This health service (or health care) dilemma is part of a wider economic problem that characterises every area of society and affects individuals, organisations, communities, societies, economies and the global community. The attempts to deal with the problem in relation to health and health care, to reduce its magnitude and effects, and achieve a closer fit between the supply of services and demand for health care provision provide an underlying theme for this book. It is important to emphasise that there is no single correct answer or solution to the problem and that health economics has the ability to deliver utopia or at least move things in such a direction. Rather what is offered in this book is an attempt to provide health care professionals with an insight into what underlies health economics, and how its techniques and processes can assist in the highly complex and emotive decisions that have to be made in health care at every hour of every day.

We all realise that there are only 24 hour in each day, that every week contains only 7 days and we do not have enough time to fit in everything that we need to do and would very much like to do. In addition, our shopping lists far exceed our abilities to purchase everything they contain, while our good intentions to maintain our strict exercise routines are often thwarted by the lack of energy after a busy day at the office, in surgery or in theatre. The fundamental economic problem is that while we all have unlimited wants and desires, we only have limited resources (time, energy, expertise and money) at our disposal to satisfy them. This situation has become particularly evident in health care and has been compounded by factors such as the increasing expectations of the population in relation to what can actually be delivered by health care services, the continuing advancements in health technology and medical science, and the increasing health needs and demands of an ageing population. For example, in the UK the number of people aged 80 and over will virtually double over the next 25 years or so, increasing from around 2.5 million (4% of population) in 2005 to nearly 5 million by 2031 (7.6% of population) and to 11% of the population by 2071. In contrast, the number of people in the working-age population in 2005 stands at 38 million (64% of total) but is set to fall to 59% of the total by 2031 (38 million) and 57% of the total in 2071 (37 million).[4]

In terms of health expenditure in the UK, for example, £67.2 billion was spent on the National Health Service (NHS) in 2002, equivalent to £1200 per person, compared to £3 billion 30 years ago, which was equivalent to £58 per person. There are now over 1.2 million employees in the NHS, a figure which has doubled over 40 years.[5] The additional resources have reaped their rewards, witnessed, for example, by the improvements in life expectancy, as shown in Figure 1.1. Males born in 1950 were expected to live for 67.7 years and women born in that year were expected to live until they were 71.8 years. By 2020, males born in that year are expected to live until they are 78.6 and females until they are 83.3.[5]

However, it should be remembered that *more* does not necessarily mean *better* health care, and diverting additional resources into health care facilities and services will not automatically generate an improvement in the health of the population. Despite increases in both the level and proportion of public expenditure devoted to the provision of health care within the UK in recent years, one of the government's influential advisers wrote (ironically in a report to the Treasury rather than the Department of Health) that 'the burden of chronic disease is growing and threatens to overwhelm the NHS . . . smoking rates must be halved during the next 20 years, and the problems of obesity and health inequalities must be tackled now if the main threats to our future health are to be avoided'.[6]

The issue of whether health care and the availability of health care facilities are the most important determinants in securing good health for society has

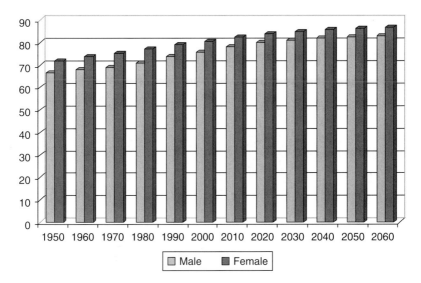

Figure 1.1 Life expectancy at birth, 1950–2060.

been widely challenged.[7–10] For instance, it has been stated that 'a society that spends so much on health care that it cannot spend adequately on other health-enhancing activities may actually be reducing the health of its popu-lation,'[8] and the issue of whether resources are used in the most beneficial way has also been raised,[9] with the suggestion that up to 25% of all health care services provided may be unnecessary.[10] Other work has demonstrated that 10–15% of health care interventions are known to reduce health status – with a similar percentage known to improve health status, and the residual 70–80% having insufficient evidence to determine their effectiveness.[11] The recent emphasis attached to evidence-based medicine and evidence-based health care has, in all probability, reduced the size of this residual, but efforts need to be maintained to ensure that the momentum in the right direction is maintained.[12,13] However, what is of concern is that a recent study under-taken by the Office of National Statistics revealed that the NHS may be wasting as much as £6 billion a year as a black hole of rising inefficiency consumes as much as 9% of the extra cash being pumped into the service, with 'tumbling productivity' accounting for much of this gap between expenditure and outputs.[14]

Another facet to consider is whether the distribution of any additional resources provided for health care services could be regarded as being fair. An increase of resources may simply reinforce existing inequalities and inequities between groups within society, and do nothing to reduce differ-ences between them in terms of life expectancy, health status or access to treatments and facilities.

This book aims to demonstrate the relevance and importance of health economics to all professionals in the health care system. It is not meant as a 'cookbook' or 'how-to-do-it manual', but rather an attempt to stimulate and challenge thinking and behaviour, and enable professionals to take on board the challenge thrown down by one of the leading health economists, Alan Williams (Professor of Health Economics, University of York), who suggested that 'in a system with limited resources, health professionals have a duty to establish not only that they are doing good, but that they are doing *more* good than anything else that could be done with the same resources'.[15]

What is economics?

As hinted above, the discipline of economics is founded on the premise that there will never be enough resources to completely satisfy human desires, referred to by economists as *scarcity*. This concept is fundamental to everything else in economics. Its importance was highlighted in an introductory chapter in a health economics textbook, which stated that 'our starting text is simply, "In the beginning, middle and end was, is and will be scarcity of resources"'.[16] As a result, the use of resources in one area inevitably means that they are not available for use in other areas, and the benefits that would have been derived from their use in other areas are sacrificed. As individuals we are constantly making choices as to how we allocate our time, into which activities we channel our energies and on what we spend our available funds. In other words, we are making *choices*. On some occasions the choices that are made at the individual level may appear, at least, rather strange (see Box 1.1), and it has been argued that we suffer from choice overload in some areas (see Box 1.2).

Box 1.1 Strange Choices

Bernard Levin, described as an influential newspaper columnist and controversialist, and as one of the two or three most influential British journalists of the late twentieth century in his obituary in *The Independent* (10 August 2004), provided an illuminating insight into the choices people make. In an article entitled 'Relative Values' in *The Times* on 27 June 1983, he highlighted the problem being faced by Copeland Council in Cumbria, England. One half of the Council's housing tenants had failed to pay their rent, which had left the Council with a major deficiency. Enquiries were made as to why people had chosen not to pay their rent and two examples of responses were provided by Levin. One family indicated that they could not afford to pay despite the main breadwinner earning £7500 a year, because they were paying £25 per week to hire five television sets and three video recorders! Another family could not pay because of the cost of their holiday to Algeria – which they had taken since it had rained every day on their earlier holiday to Malta!

> **Box 1.2 Take Your Choice**
>
> When we were lads, we'd go over to the bakers for a loaf of bread, and there'd be a choice of brown or white. If you were lucky, you might have a choice of sliced or unsliced. Butter? Well, you could have butter or Stork margarine.
>
> Or take something as simple as shampoo. Time was when it was just shampoo. Then it was shampoo for dry, normal or greasy hair. Cool. Then it was for permed or fly-away hair. Cooler still. Then anti-dandruff. Seems a good idea. Then for hair that's been in the sun too long. OK, I'm still with you. Or especially for blonde hair; now I'm beginning to get just a little bit cynical: how can washing blonde hair be any different from washing brown hair? There's shampoo for hair with split ends – presumably containing glue to stick the ends back together. Shampoo for hair that's been dyed, and shampoo [for hair] that's been dyed and is returning to normal. There's shampoo for highlighted hair and for low-lighted hair. Shampoo for thick or frizzy hair. And that's not to mention 'wash and go'. The shampoo shelves in the supermarket used to have about three varieties across 6 inches of shelf space. Now it's about 6 feet across and five shelves deep and it takes you half an hour to find the one you want.
>
> We are plagued by the tyranny of choice.
>
> *Source*: Bill Bryson. In Preeble S (ed). *Grumpy Old Men*. London: BBC Books, 2004: 124–26.

In addition, governments also provide examples of confused thinking, at best. Billions of pounds are spent each year on the NHS to improve health and prevent death, while at the same time so-called scarce resources are being poured into manufacturing bombs and developing military hardware in order to maim and kill people! Another example of a 'lack of joined-up policy-making' was illustrated in the government's response to a series of railway crashes. The Hatfield railway crash in October 2000, following on from two other serious railway crashes near London, had brought about a series of headlines in the press crying out for something to be done about the apparent lack of safety and risk to rail passengers within the UK. In contrast, the headline in *The Economist* was that 'Britain spends too much money, not too little, making its railways safe'[17] and that 'overreaction to last month's rail crash has increased the risks to rail passengers, not reduced them'.[18] It concluded:

> From society's point of view it is far from rational to spend 150 times as much on saving a life on the railways as on saving a life on the roads. A bereaved mother cares little how her child was killed. Many more lives could be saved if the money currently being poured into avoiding

spectacular but rare railway crashes were spent instead on avoiding the tragedies that happen ten times every day on the roads.[17]

It is therefore very apparent that in making a choice to spend our time on one activity or purchase a certain commodity means that period of time and those funds are not available for other activities and for other purchases. As a result, the benefits that would have been derived are sacrificed. These sacrifices are referred to as *opportunity cost*. Their very existence provides a rationale for economists to take an interest in all resources that are used, whether by individuals, governments, the health service or society, regardless of whether or not money is paid for them, in order to achieve the maximum benefit for society.

Questions of resource allocation, that is, how society's scarce resources are, could be or should be allocated amongst the infinite variety of competing activities, are fundamental to any study of economics. The wide range of economic systems, which have existed and evolved over time, have all attempted to address the basic economic problem of allocating resources in such a way as to maximise the benefits for society. Similarly, the varieties of approaches employed to fund and finance health care by different countries all have the same basic aim – of seeking to maximise the health benefits for their citizens, given the resources they have available at that point of time. The issue of whether governments should exercise more control over their respective economies or whether the market mechanism should be allowed to operate freely has exercised the minds of economists over many centuries, and the extent of governmental involvement in economic decision-making continues to stimulate debate in policy circles, academic institutions, the media and other popular centres of debate and discussion.

In the UK the creation of the NHS in 1945 took place at a time when economic policy was undergoing a fundamental change, where the government took a more active role in determining how resources were to be allocated, and adopting the policies advocated by John Maynard Keynes. He had argued that governments could introduce appropriate policies to counter the swings of boom and bust, to which the economy had been subjected, and which led to the great depression and mass unemployment levels of the 1920s and 1930s. The government could intervene in the economy to avoid the consequences associated with unemployment by increasing levels of public expenditure or reducing taxation, while if there was danger that the economy was overheating, they could impose restrictive measures designed to dampen the levels of demand and activity. The post-war Labour government was in favour of such policies and introduced a very radical programme. During this period, a number of industries were nationalised and brought under the control of the State, which, at the same time, determined levels of employment and production. These policies were implemented by successive UK governments until the mid- to late 1970s, when a series of significant economic problems combined to bring the UK economy to a crisis. During the mid-1970s as well, the thinking in the Conservative Party had changed and an entirely different perspective of the operation of the economy was being promulgated, known as Monetarism, based on the work of Milton Freedman and others. The new leader of the Conservative Party, Margaret Thatcher, had embraced these ideas, and when her government was elected in 1979, it summoned another watershed in UK economic policy. Shares in industries, which for more than 30 years had been under state control, were sold and the drive for privatisation began. Thatcher was committed to 'rolling back the frontiers of the public sector' and her aim was to give the 'market' a greater say in determining the economic prosperity of the nation. It appeared that no industry or service was exempt from this drive and, in 1989, the NHS found itself subject to the influence of the market, with the establishment of the so-called Internal Market, in the government White Paper entitled 'Working for Patients'.[19] Many of the ideas contained in the White Paper were based on the work of Alain Enthoven[20] and revolved around the notion that money flows would follow patients and that 'purchasers' of services would place contracts with those 'providers' deemed to be the most successful and best able to meet their requirements.

The market, in economic terms, comprises a *demand* side – based on consumers' wants and desires, supported by an ability to pay for the particular commodity, and a *supply* side – based on producers' aim to generate profit, and the interaction between them. Markets operate according to price signals, that is, if prices change, demand and supply will adjust to a position where producers will be able to sell all that they want at that price, and consumers will be able to purchase all that they want at that particular price. Similarly, if levels of demand and/or supply alter, the price will adjust to reflect such changes and move to a position where demand and supply are again equal. Proponents of the market system believe that its 'invisible hand' will result in an allocation of resources that will maximise the benefits to society, known as *Pareto-efficiency*, named after, and based on the work of, the Italian sociologist of the nineteenth century.

While the objective of endeavouring to maximise the benefits to society, given the level of resources available, appears at first sight to be perfectly valid and commendable, there are a number of other issues that impinge on the pursuit of such an objective. For example, it has been stated that 'as efficient as markets may be, they do not ensure that individuals have enough food, clothes to wear, or shelter'.[21] In an extreme case, the market mechanism might result in all resources being allocated to a few individuals within society, with everyone else receiving nothing. Such a situation is obviously unacceptable and, in reality, it is impossible to separate decisions regarding resource allocation from those regarding income distribution. To ensure that resource allocation and income distribution are considered, there has to be a degree of 'external involvement' – usually governmental – in the operation of the market to counter such extreme scenarios from developing. What remains an issue is the extent of such government involvement.

These two issues are vitally important in economics and together they combine to form, what has been termed, the social welfare function, with its individual components of efficiency and equity. In constructing policy decisions there is a broad consensus that both of these aspects of social welfare should be considered in the location, method and degree of government intervention in health care, and there is general agreement that there is a need for a trade-off between achieving an efficient allocation of resources and ensuring that the resulting allocation is equitable. However, in recent years, economic pressures and political imperatives have tended to result in governments focusing more on efficiency as the main driving force in formulating health care policy.

The notion of efficiency

The term *efficiency* is used by economists to consider the extent to which decisions relating to the allocation of limited resources maximises the benefits for society and has been defined as 'maximising well-being at the least cost to society'.[22] The concept of efficiency embraces inputs (costs) and outputs and/or outcomes (benefits) and the relationship between them, with a society being judged in efficiency terms by the extent to which it maximises the benefits for its population, given the resources at its disposal. The simplest notion of efficiency is the one synonymous with economy, and is often referred to as *efficiency savings*, where output is expected to be maintained, while at the same time making cost reductions, or where additional output is generated with the same level of inputs. This type of efficiency has been referred to as technical efficiency[23] or operational efficiency,[22,24] but also as cost-effectiveness.[22,25,26] It is applied where a choice needs to be made between alternatives that seek to achieve the same goal, and exists when output is maximised for a given cost, or where the costs of producing a given output are minimised. It is widely used in the context where, for example, new therapies are compared against existing treatments, and authorities have to decide whether it is worth paying more for the potential additional benefits that the new therapy offers.

However, technical efficiency or cost-effectiveness is not sufficient in order to establish priorities, both within health care systems and when comparing the provision of health care with other publicly funded services. In order to determine whether and how certain services should be provided, and in order to establish priorities, allocative efficiency must be used. This type of efficiency exists when it is impossible to make one person better off without at the same time making someone else worse off. It represents a situation where no input and no output can be transferred so as to make someone better off without at the same time making someone else worse off. This situation is called *Pareto-efficient*, referred to above.

However, in reality, there may well be situations where a reallocation of resources would result in some people being made better off while others would be worse off. It is possible that there could be a net overall improvement if the beneficiaries were to compensate the losers and still be better off. This has been referred to as *social efficiency* and such a situation exists when 'there is no scope for potential Pareto improvement'.[23] An example of social efficiency is discussed in Box 1.3.

Box 1.3 The Weekend in Paris Principle!

Post-operative nausea and vomiting (PONV) is a common complication associated with anaesthesia and surgery, with 20–30% of surgical patients suffering from the symptoms. It can cause significant patient discomfort and, in out-patient procedures, may result in readmission or delay discharge and require the diversion of additional resources to deal with the problems. Drugs that reduce the incidence and frequency of PONV are available but the decision of whether to utilise such drugs as a preventive strategy or as a form of treatment remains somewhat inconclusive. Almost 40 years ago it was suggested that it may be better to see who vomits and then treat. On the other hand, is it acceptable to wait and see if a patient vomits or becomes nauseated before starting a treatment?

It has been shown that, in the case of ondansetron, a 5HT3-receptor antagonist, it is cost-effective to adopt the wait- and-see treatment strategy rather than the prophylactic approach. However, the outcomes resulting from prophylactic and treatment strategies are not the same and consideration needs to be given to the nature, magnitude and value attached to such differences. If there is a change in policy away from prophylaxis to treatment, a situation emerges where some patients will be made better off while others would be worse off. The 'losers' would be patients who suffer a PONV episode but would not have done so if they had been given the drug as a prophylactic, while the 'gainers' would be the anaesthetics department whose budgetary position has been improved by the switch in policy. The question thus emerges – by how much can these departments 'compensate' the 'losers' and still emerge with budgetary improvements?

On the basis of the cost-effectiveness calculations, and if prophylaxis was the norm, the extent of potential 'savings' available as a result of a change to treatment would range from £20 to over £200 per successfully treated patient – and, in an age of relatively cheap flights, a weekend in Paris!! When these amounts are extended across the number of people who are given prophylactic interventions to prevent PONV on an annual basis, they constitute significant sums of money and percentages of health organisations' budgets.

Source: Based on Tramèr *et al.* [27]

As indicated earlier, it is impossible to separate the drive towards an efficient allocation of resources from its impact on income distribution. A move towards Pareto-efficiency may well result in a redistribution of income in favour of the well off, which may not be acceptable on grounds of fairness and equity.

The notion of equity

Virtually all health care systems employ a mix of libertarian and egalitarian values, that is, a combination of services provided by market forces and those controlled and regulated by the government. Even within the US system, which places considerable emphasis on the role of the market in health care, there are two major insurance schemes, one for the elderly (Medicare) and one for poorer members of society (Medicaid). The notion of equity is inextricably linked with notions of fairness and justice, but it is important to distinguish it from the concept of equality, which is the 'condition of being equal' (*Oxford English Dictionary*). Policies designed to achieve equality of opportunity, or access, or utilisation or outcome may well be desirous but they need not necessarily be equitable. One of the leading exponents of libertarian thinking, Frederick Hayeck, argued that 'as a statement of fact, it is not just true that "all men are born equal" . . . and if we treat them equally, the result must be inequality in their actual position'.[28] Donaldson and Gerard highlighted the problems in arriving at what they regard as the unobtainable 'gold standard' of equality of health,[24] and suggested that the focus of policies should be on equality relating to health care rather than health. It is useful here to distinguish between *horizontal equity* and *vertical equity*. The former refers to the 'equal treatment of equals' and the latter to the 'unequal treatment of unequals'.[16] In other words, a programme would be regarded as equitable if 'similar outcomes were achieved for people with similar needs' but inequitable and unjust if 'similar services were provided for people with different needs'.[3,29]

In terms of horizontal equity the issue is whether the reference point is equal resources (expenditure), or opportunity, or utilisation or access for equal need. However, whichever perspective is employed, the actual achievement of it in practice is extremely difficult.[24,29] Despite these conceptual problems, the extent of health inequalities within countries and across international boundaries continues to ensure that equity remains high on the list of health policy objectives. Many influential national and international policy documents highlight the importance of equity as a goal of policy and the ongoing need to implement remedial measures to reduce inequalities both between and within populations, which remain frustratingly large. A recent commentary on attempts to address health inequalities within the UK highlighted the misconceptions surrounding inequalities and inequities and the complexity of dealing with them.[30] It demonstrated the danger of selective reporting of statistics and emphasised the need to place the alleviation of inequalities alongside other health-related policy objectives in the context of an ethical framework, to determine which inequalities actually constitute inequities, and the opportunity costs involved in attempting to reduce the extent of such inequalities. It is clear that there is no consensus as to the type of policies and processes required in order to achieve such goals. Should policies be designed to ensure that those who have made a 'positive' contribution to society receive a greater share of benefits than those who have made a 'negative' contribution? Should more benefits be received by those on whom many others depend rather than those on whom nobody depends?[31] No one, for example, would advocate encouraging people in higher socioeconomic groups to engage in health-damaging behaviour, such as increasing their levels and rates of smoking, to reduce their health status and as a consequence reduce inequalities in health across social groups!

An issue that has really polarised opinion, both within the health care professions and among decision-makers, for example, is whether people who knowingly engage in health-damaging behaviour should receive treatment – is it fair and equitable that limited health care resources are allocated to these people, while others, who have attempted to live healthy lives, have to wait for treatment or access the services of the private sector? The very fact that service provision is limited makes it inevitable that some people will not receive all that is wanted or even required. The decision-making process as to who should receive services, treatments and interventions is littered with casualties, who can legitimately claim that such decisions are unfair and inequitable. In addition, there is a lack of consensus on how to deal with policies that improve efficiency while increasing inequalities, or those that improve fairness while decreasing efficiency.[32] The National Institute for Clinical Excellence (NICE) was launched in the UK following the disapproval of the 'postcode-prescribing' lottery, which had existed as different health authorities formulated different policies on which treatments they would fund. NICE has been expressly concerned with identifying clinically effective and cost-effective technologies 'to remove unfairness in the availability of technologies in different localities and to minimise the possibility of further examples of unfairness or inequity being introduced'.[33] However, the implementation of NICE recommendations may not necessarily result in an improvement in efficiency or remove inequities of access and provision.[34–36] Without additional funding, the NHS, at a local level, must deny funding to other services in order to finance NICE recommendations, since it is a requirement that new treatments approved by NICE have to be funded within 3 months of the decision[37] – thereby achieving greater equity in some areas of service provision at the expense of creating inequities in others.

It is widely acknowledged that people's environment, social status, educational achievements, ethical origin, age, gender, etc. affect their state of health, and equally that their conditions and characteristics result in some being better able to respond to treatments and enjoy longer life expectancy.[22] For example, life expectancy rates exhibit wide variation across the UK. Males born in Glasgow have a life expectancy of 69.1 years, while those born in

East Dorset can expect to live for 11 years longer.[38] However, these rates are put into stark perspective when compared with life expectancy in some of the developing countries. For example, the life expectancy in Ghana is 57.6 years, while in Côte d'Ivoire it is 45.3 and in Angola it is 39.9 years.[39]

The influential Health Commission, also known as the Commission for Health Care Audit and Inspection (CHAI), was launched on 1 April 2004 to promote improvement in the quality of health care within England and Wales. It replaced (but encapsulated many of its roles and objectives) the Commission for Health Improvement, which had been set up in 1999 to drive forward the government's quality agenda and secure *fair access for all*. One of the consequences of the agenda for quality improvements was the introduction of additional targets. As a result, hospitals are faced with inspection and assessment overload brought about as a result of over 100 organisations with the power to inspect UK hospitals and each requiring information and statistics to help them fulfil their responsibilities.[40] In its first report, CHAI announced that 'there are variations in health across difference ethnic groups: diabetes, for example, is six times more common among South Asians. There are differences in people's experiences of health service: for example, it is striking that compulsory admissions to mental health units appear to be disproportionately high for some black and minority ethnic groups. There are also inconsistencies in the provision of services: for example, the proportion of older people receiving flu vaccinations varies from 78% to 49% across primary care trusts.''[41]

The Audit Commission also reported on the differentials across the country in terms of service provision and commented that some populations have 'no local access to services for patients with long-lasting pain'.[42] Unless remedial measures are introduced it is likely that such situations will deteriorate, as demographic factors intensify the demand for chronic pain services for the foreseeable future, at least.[43]

It is therefore evident that in setting the economic objectives of health care systems, both efficiency and equity considerations are vital components and must be given serious consideration.[24] However, it is inevitable that in seeking to achieve a more equitable allocation of resources, a level of efficiency will have to be sacrificed, or, in attempting to move to a more efficient health care system, inequalities in provision or access to services may have to be compromised. For example, the overall health benefits to society, in terms of lives saved and events avoided, of locating an open access chest pain clinic in a hospital serving a large urban area is likely to be much greater than if it were placed in a smaller rural hospital with a much smaller population base. However, what such a decision also does is to reinforce the inequalities in provision, access and probably outcome between urban and rural areas. Reversing the decision would obviously reduce such inequalities but at the cost of an overall deterioration in quality of life (QOL) and increases in the numbers of lives lost.

What is health economics?

The two concepts of efficiency and equity lie at the heart of the discipline of health economics. In simple terms health economics has been described as the discipline of economics applied to the topic of health,[16] or as 'a logical and explicit framework to aid health care workers, decision-makers, governments, or society at large, to make choices on how best to use resources'.[44]

As indicated earlier, the relationship between expenditure on health care services and the health status of a population is not directly proportional. It is far too simplistic to argue that in order to improve the health of the nation and reduce inequalities additional resources need to be channelled into health care services. The USA spends approximately 14% of its gross domestic product (GDP) on health care, over 2.5 times the average health expenditure of the other 29 OECD (Organization for Economic Cooperation and Development) countries, but is one of the least healthy of these nations, being ranked 21st out of 30 in terms of life expectancy. Japan, which spends about 7% of its GDP on health care, is one of the healthiest with a life expectancy of nearly 82 years – 4 years greater than the USA.[45] In addition, it has been shown that there is a level of health care expenditure where maximum benefits are being produced and beyond which extra health gains cease to exist, and patients may actually be harmed. This has been termed 'flat of the curve' practice and many examples of this type of practice have been highlighted.[22,46]

Understanding the state of health within a nation and differences between communities in relation to their health status requires thinking about the determinants of health,[47] which include not only the quality and quantity of health care facilities available but also the level of education, state of the housing stock, nutrition and diet of the population, and economic state of the nation and its citizens.

Since Adam Smith published *The Wealth of Nations* in 1776, the relationship between economic productivity and the health of society has been recognised. Longitudinal studies, with a range of designs, provide reasonably good evidence that unemployment itself is detrimental to health and has an impact on health outcomes – increasing mortality rates, causing physical and mental ill health and greater use of health services.[48] However, it is not clear as to what is cause and what is effect. Is it the case that those with relatively poor health face a greater risk of becoming unemployed? Does unemployment itself cause deterioration in health? The direction of causality is one which has tended to dominate the debate in the literature, and the issue has been expanded further by questions that ask whether the association between unemployment and health arises because of the link between unemployment and poverty, or because both unemployment and poor health are related to other factors, such as poorer education, lower socioeconomic status and worse housing conditions. People at the lower end of the social spectrum generally are in poorer health, have lower life expectancies and have higher utilisation rates than those at the other end. The inequalities in health as a result of social status were highlighted by two highly influential reports in the 1980s – the Black Report[49] and the Health Divide.[50] The reports provided concrete examples to support the claims that poverty was a major factor in determining who was affected by the killer diseases and who suffered greater levels of chronic sickness. It was apparent that children living in poverty tended to have lower birth weights, shorter stature and were more likely to suffer from high prevalence of tooth decay. What was also evident was that these major inequalities were evident between adjacent communities in the same region, with affluent communities enjoying good health, while areas suffering from social and material deprivation experiencing very poor health. For example, the percentage of people in one unitary authority area in Wales, Monmouthshire, which reported having long-term illness, was under 30, while in the neighbouring authority, Blaenau Gwent, the percentage was over 40.[51]

In general terms it can be argued that the health service has been a victim of its own success. Reference was made earlier to the improvements in life expectancy, while infant mortality rates in the UK have fallen from over 30 per 1000 live births in 1950 to 5 per 1000 live births at present.[5] Contrary to what had been thought at the inception of the NHS – that as the population's health improved the demands placed on health care services would diminish – the opposite has been the case and the demands that are placed on health care services are consistently rising despite improvements in the health of communities. People living longer with higher expectations, technological advancements and developments in medical science have resulted in a health care system that is way beyond the wildest dreams of the founders of the NHS. However, as the nature of health care problems experienced by the population has changed, the costs of developing treatment and care pro-grammes to deal with such problems have continued to increase. The level of resources available to fund such services has not increased to the same extent, and we are therefore left with the dilemma of how to allocate limited resources to meet the demands placed on the health services and maximise the health care benefit to society.

The nature of the health care dilemma, which confronts virtually all health care systems, is depicted in Figure 1.2.[1–3] It is a microcosm of the basic economic problem that confronts all individuals, organisations and societies – that of reconciling infinite wants, needs and demands with finite resource availability, in terms of income, time, expertise and so on. The exponential increase in the demand for health care services has been occurring at the same time as pressures on governments and funding agencies to carefully manage the volume of resources available for health care services.

Obviously, additional resources would help, but even if expenditure on health care services (measured by the proportion of GDP allocated to health care) matched that of other countries, the gap between demand and supply would still be enormous. In addition, the question then has to be asked as to

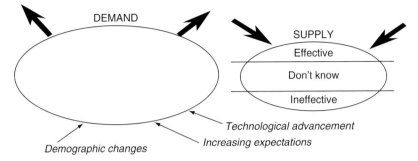

Figure 1.2 The health care dilemma.

which area(s) of health care the additional funds should be allocated to. For example, additional resources for cancer services would mean that these resources are not available for use in, for example, coronary heart disease. Similarly, decisions on where additional resources should be allocated need to be made with information relating to the effectiveness of interventions, the competence of health care professionals and the safety of health care facilities. The need for evidence on the effectiveness of interventions has resulted in something of an evangelistic campaign, over the past 10 years or so, to ensure that clinical decisions are based on evidence of what works and what does not. In addition, the social status of doctors in society has shifted from that of experts, whose judgement was to be trusted and who were left to carry out their duties relatively unchallenged at the beginning of the twentieth century, to the current situation, where levels of public trust have been severely diluted as a result of high-profile media cases, but also as an increasingly educated, informed and questioning public has sought reassurance that public finances are being used efficiently.[52]

Irrespective, therefore, of the level of resources that are made available, choices will still have to be made. The choices that have to be made in health care are not between holidays and kitchens, for example, but whether additional resources should be made available for geriatrics or paediatrics or diabetes or gastroenterology or mental health. Other choices have to be made in specific disease areas. For example, should additional resources be provided to fund the further development of cardiac units or to increase the proportion of the population receiving cholesterol-lowering, statin therapy or to construct and implement effective smoking-cessation programmes? Who is to decide these issues? How can these choices be made? In the arena of health care, such choices can have profound and devastating consequences. As Professor Alan Williams, Health Economist at University of York, stated: 'I believe that being efficient is a moral obligation, not a managerial convenience, for not to be efficient means imposing avoidable death and unnecessary suffering on people who might have benefited from the resources which are being used wastefully.'[53]

Health care professionals are increasingly being exposed to extremely powerful and emotive choices, and in no way can health economics provide the solution to such complex and difficult issues. What it does offer is a mode of thinking that can assist in arriving at possible solutions (notice the use of the term 'assist' here – health economics cannot by itself offer the solutions, it has to be part of a wide-ranging approach to decision-making) to these often contentious problems. It aims to identify which package or bundle of services would provide the maximum health care benefit for society within the envelope of resources available. It is the same process as we go through as individuals, in making that decision between a holiday abroad or a new kitchen – the first will provide us with significant benefits within a short period of time but the duration of these will soon diminish as we return to our normal existence. The kitchen, on the other hand, will provide fewer benefits immediately in comparison, but the duration of the benefits will extend for a number of years. The prices of the alternatives are basically the same but we can only afford one of them. What factors do we consider in making the decision? How do we go about making these difficult choices? How do we decide which programmes and projects to fund? The use of health economics techniques can help in making these decisions but they should always be just one part of a multifaceted process, with other factors also being considered.

In our more rational moments we would try and weigh up what we will get in terms of benefits for the amount of money we spend on our new kitchen or holiday. It is basically the same process when we apply economics to health care. What do we get in terms of health care benefits for the resources we put in?

In order to address these questions there are a number of issues that need to be grappled with. We need to know what level of resources is needed to fund certain programmes and interventions. In other words, we need to determine the costs of provision. This is far from being straightforward and more attention is devoted to this in Chapter 3. We then need to know what we get from the resources we put in. It is relatively straightforward to quantify the number of patients who pass through the surgery or have been treated, but such an approach does not tell us their condition, or their health state post intervention as compared with that prior to the intervention, etc. We need perhaps to adopt the policy to measure what is important rather than making important what we measure. We also have to endeavour to develop common currencies so that apples and pears can be compared – that is, outputs and outcomes in obstetrics and gynaecology need to be compared with outputs and outcomes in renal disease, care of the elderly, musculoskeletal disorders, etc. These issues are addressed in more detail in Chapter 4. In Chapter 5 the costs of health care interventions and services are brought together with the outputs and outcomes resulting from these services and interventions, and attention is focused on what is meant by economic evaluation, or what has conventionally (but not strictly or accurately) been referred to as cost-effectiveness. Chapter 6 explores the role of health economics in decision-making in more detail, while Chapter 7, the final chapter, considers some of the future challenges facing health services and health professionals, and how an awareness of health economics, and the framework for thinking that it provides, can assist.

References

1 Phillips CJ, Prowle MJ. Evaluating a health campaign: the Heartbeat Wales no-smoking initiative. *Contemp Wales* 1992; 5: 187–212.
2 Phillips CJ. Cost-effectiveness of anaesthesia and analgesia, in Tramèr MR (ed). *Evidence-based resource in anaesthesia and analgesia.* London: BMJ Books, 2003.
3 Palfrey C, Thomas P, Phillips CJ. *Effective healthcare management: an evaluative approach.* Oxford: Blackwell, 2004.
4 Office of National Statistics. *http://www.statistics.gov.uk/downloads/theme-population/PP2No24.pdf* (accessed 17 January 2005)
5 Office of Health Economics. *Compendium of health statistics.* London: Office of Health Economics, 2002.
6 Wanless D. Securing good health for the whole population. HM Treasury, 2004. *http://www.hm-treasury.gov.uk./media/E43/27/Wanless04_summary.pdf* (accessed 12 January 2004)
7 Edwards RT. Paradigms and research programmes: is it time to move from health care economics to health economics. *Health Econ* 2001; 10: 635–49.
8 Evans RG, Stoddart GL. Producing health, consuming health care, in Evans RG, Barer ML, Marmor TRE (eds). *Why are some people healthy and others are not? The determinants of health of populations.* New York: Aldine de Gruyter, 1994.
9 Moore A. Waste in the NHS: the problem, its size and how we can tackle it. *Bandolier Extra* 2002. *http://www.jr2.ox.ac.uk/bandolier/Extraforbando/Waste.pdf* (accessed 16 October 2004)
10 Borowitz M, Sheldon T. Controlling health care: from economic interventions to micro-clinical regulation. *Health Econ* 1993; 2: 201–204.
11 Warner M, Evans W. Pearls of wisdom. *Health Serv J* 1993; September 16: 20–21.
12 Walshe K. Evidence-based policy: don't be timid. *BMJ* 2001; 323: 187.
13 Donald A. Research must be taken seriously. *BMJ* 2001; 323: 278–79.
14 Office of National Statistics. *Public service productivity: health.* Paper 1. *http://www.statistics.gov.uk/cci/article.asp?id=987* (accessed 20 October 2004)
15 Williams A speaking at Healthy Outcomes Conference, 16 September 1993 and reported in MacLachlan R, Glasman D. A case of myth management. *Health Service Journal* 1993; 103(5370): 12–13.
16 Mooney G. *Economics, medicine and health care.* London: Harvester Wheatsheaf, 1992.
17 The Economist. The price of safety. *The Economist* 2000; 357(8198): 23.
18 The Economist. How not to run a railway. *The Economist* 2000; 357(8198): 35–36.
19 Department of Health. *Working for patients.* London: HMSO, 1989.
20 Enthoven A. *Reflections on the management of the NHS.* London: Nuffield Provincial Hospitals Trust, 1985.
21 Stiglitz JE. *Globalization and its discontents.* London: Penguin Books, 2002.
22 Mitton G, Donaldson C. *Priority setting toolkit: a guide to the use of economics in healthcare decision making.* London: BMJ Books, 2004.

23 McGuire A, Henderson J. *The economics of health care: an introductory text*. London: Routledge and Kegan Paul, 1987.

24 Donaldson C, Gerard K. *Economics of health care financing: the visible hand*. Basingstoke: Macmillan, 1993.

25 Gerard K. Cost-utility in practice: a policy maker's guide to the state of the art. *Health Policy* 1992; 21: 249–79.

26 Drummond MF, O'Brien B, Stoddart GL *et al*. *Methods for the economic evaluation of healthcare programmes*. Oxford: Oxford University Press, 1997.

27 Tramèr MR, Phillips CJ, Reynolds DJM *et al*. Cost-effectiveness of ondansetron for postoperative nausea and vomiting. *Anaesthesia* 1999; 54: 226–34.

28 Hayek F. *The constitution of liberty*. London: Routledge and Kegan Paul, 1960.

29 Phillips CJ, Palfrey CF, Thomas P. *Evaluating health and social care*. Basingstoke: Macmillan, 1994.

30 Oliver A, Healey A, Le Grand J. Addressing health inequalities. *Lancet* 2002; 360: 565–67.

31 Williams A. Beyond effectiveness and efficiency . . . lies equality! in Maynard A, Chalmers I (eds). *Non-random reflections on health services research: on the 25th anniversary of Archie Cochrane's 'Effectiveness and Efficiency'*. London: BMJ Books, 1997.

32 Sassi F, Le Grand J, Archard L. Equity versus efficiency: a dilemma for the NHS. *BMJ* 2001; 323: 762–63.

33 National Institute for Clinical Excellence. *Technical guidance for manufacturers and sponsors on making a submission to a technology appraisal*. London: National Institute for Clinical Excellence, 2001.

34 Doyle Y. Equity in the new NHS: hard lessons from implementing a local healthcare policy on donepezil. *BMJ* 2001; 323: 222–24.

35 Burke K. No cash to implement NICE, health authorities tell MPs. *BMJ* 2002; 324: 258.

36 Smith R. The failings of NICE. *BMJ* 2000; 321: 1363–64.

37 Dent THS, Sadler M. From guidance to practice: why NICE is not enough. *BMJ* 2002; 324: 842–45.

38 Office of National Statistics. *Life expectancy at birth by health and local authorities in the United Kingdom*. 1991–1993 to 1999–2001 – revised figures using 2001 census based population estimates. *http://www.statistics.gov.uk/downloads/theme_population/Life_Expect_Birth_UK_1991–93_1999–01.pdf* (accessed 26 February 2004)

39 WHO. *World Health Report 2004: statistical annex. http://www.who.int/whr/2004/annex/topic/en/annex_1_en.pdf* (accessed 17 January 2005)

40 Lister S. Hospitals tied up by 102 red-tape visitors. *The Times* 9 October 2004: 14.

41 Health Commission. *State of Healthcare Report 2004. http://www.chai.org.uk/assetRoot/04/00/63/66/04006366.pdf* (accessed 20 December 2004)

42 Audit Commission. *Anaesthesia under examination*. London: Audit Commission, 1997.

43 McQuay HJ, Moore RA, Eccleston C *et al*. Systematic review of outpatient services for chronic patient control. *Health Tech Assess* 1997; 1(6).

44 Jefferson T, Demicheli V, Mugford M. *Elementary economic evaluation in health care*. London: BMJ Books, 2000.

45 Gould E. *Health care: US spends more, gets less*. Economic Policy Institute Snapshots. *http://www.epinet.org/content.cfm/webfeatures_snapshots_10202004* (accessed 21 December 2004)

46 Mallenson A. *Whiplash and other useful illnesses*. Montreal: McGill-Queen's University Press, 2002.

47 Evans RG, Stoddart GL. Producing health, consuming health care. *Soc Sci Med* 1990; 31: 1347–63.

48 Mathers CD, Schofield DJ. The health consequences of unemployment: the evidence. *Med J Aust* 1998; 168(4): 178–82.

49 Department of Health and Social Security. *Inequalities in health: report of a research working group chaired by Sir Douglas Black*. London: HMSO, 1980.

50 Whitehead M. *The health divide*. London: Health Education Council, 1987.

51 National Assembly for Wales. *Welsh Health Survey 1998*. Cardiff: Government Statistical Service, 1999.

52 Davies HTO, Nutley SM, Smith PC. Learning from the past, prospects for the future, in Davies HTO, Nutley SM, Smith PC (eds). *What works? Evidence-based policy and practice in public services*. Bristol: The Policy Press, 2000.

53 Williams A. Ethics, clinical freedom and the doctors' role, in Culyer AJ, Maynard A, Posnett J (eds). *Competition in health care: reforming the NHS*. Basingstoke: Macmillan, 1990.

CHAPTER 2

Organisation and funding of health care services

The aims of this chapter are to outline relevant features of health care systems, with particular reference to organisation of the NHS in the UK; to identify some of the issues and problems involved in its organisation and funding; to consider the role of health care professionals and their relationships with managers and patients; and, to consider approaches to funding health care services and how much should be spent on health services.

Features of health care systems

As governments and societies attempt to maximise the level of health care benefits generated from the resources available, the nature of health care systems and their funding mechanisms are never far from the discussions and deliberations that take place in academic, political and professional communities. Reforms and change have been the order of the day in many health care systems and, while any attempt to assess their relative success has been virtually impossible given the frequency and extent of such developments, one common thread has appeared to be transference of decision-making to a more local level. In the UK, the reforms introduced in the early 1990s paved the way for the present situation where local decision-makers are required to establish priorities and allocate resources. The separation of the agencies that commission, organise or purchase services from those that provide health care services has become a common feature of health care reforms across many European countries.[1] As a result, patients may have to bypass their local hospitals and travel across both national and international boundaries in order to receive treatment, and NHS patients may be found in hospital beds alongside private patients, as well as the opposite scenario, which has a longer history.

The extent of private sector involvement in health care systems has been another feature in the ongoing debate about the funding and organisation of health care services. For example, just as there is greater involvement with the private sector hospitals in the UK, the Private Finance Initiative (PFI) has become the main source of capital funds for major investment projects in the

NHS, funding 85% of major capital projects since 1997.[2] However, there are major concerns as to the effectiveness and efficiency of PFI as a vehicle for building new capacity within the NHS, with counter claims suggesting that it actually constrains service provision and limits future developments, and may not actually represent value for money as originally envisaged,[3] and 'there appears to be no macroeconomic justification for preferring PFI to Exchequer financing, or for regarding one approach as any more affordable than the other'.[2]

The organisational structure of health care systems is also subject to variation and what appears to be more or less constant change and reform. In 1989 the UK Department of Health White Paper 'Working for Patients'[4] proposed a set of reforms in an attempt to improve the performance of the NHS, based on what came to be known as 'internal market'. Under the new arrangements, hospitals and community health units were designated as NHS Trusts and became the main 'providers' of front-line health services. They were required to compete with each other for contracts from Health Authorities (HAs) and general practitioner (GP) Fundholders who were established as the purchasers or 'commissioners' of services. The new organisational structure, which sought to emphasise decentralisation and entrepreneurship, ran counter to other health policy initiatives of the time, most notably The Patient's Charter and the Health of the Nation strategies, which sought to impose central standards and targets.[5] It was also argued that the experiment with a competitive quasi-market in health care for the NHS did not really succeed because in the main it was not tried, as the government was reluctant to reduce the extent of centralised control.[6,7]

It was therefore no surprise that in 1997, the new Labour government declared that the internal market and the reliance on 'competition' as the basis for improving performance in the NHS would come to an end.[8] In their place would come a return to collaboration, partnership, integration and the development of new structures to replace the existing HAs. New organisations (with different nomenclatures evident in different parts of the devolved UK) in primary care were constituted to emphasise the increasingly important role of primary care in the planning of health care and to cooperate with secondary care providers. These independent trusts control a highly significant percentage of the NHS budget and have the capability of retaining budget surpluses and utilising these for the benefit of patients in their locality.[7]

However, there remain serious capacity constraints within the NHS in the UK, particularly in terms of doctors and nurses – a problem that may intensify if some commentators are to be believed. A report in the media has suggested, for instance, that thousands of the country's most experienced doctors may quit the NHS within 3 years after the introduction of the new contract in 2005, which means they can retire early on full pensions. The new contract boosts the salaries of top consultants by £20 000 to £92 000. Their pension contributions will rise in line with their pay, meaning that they will hit the maximum achievable pension – just under half their salary – by their early sixties. Some could even retire as early as their mid-fifties with only a slight deduction in their retirement benefits. For most there will be little incentive to keep working punishing NHS schedules until mandatory retirement. The stark warning presented is that by 2007 nearly 4000 senior consultants will have little or no financial incentive to continue working for the NHS and any mass exodus would exacerbate staffing problems in the service, which at present has a shortfall of 10 000 hospital doctors.[9]

The Wanless Report estimated that an extra 30 000 doctors, 24 000 nurses and 94 000 qualified scientific, technical and ancillary workers were needed over the next 20 years or so,[10] but even this achievement would not change the position of the UK as below the EU average in the number of doctors and nurses per 1000 population.[7]

In addition, the development of league tables, the continued use of performance indicators, the establishment of 'Foundation hospitals', the ongoing political debate surrounding so-called 'patient choice', and the role and extent of involvement of the private sector in the UK make it difficult to ignore the imperative of competitiveness within the health care system. For example, in a comparison of the NHS with a health maintenance organisation in the USA, Kaiser Permanente, the latter achieved better performance at roughly the same cost as the NHS because of integration throughout the system, efficient management of hospital use, *the benefits of competition* and greater investment in information technology.[11] At the same time, the nature of the NHS and its financing continue to focus the attention of policymakers, politicians, academics and health care professionals. The rationale for government involvement in the organisation and funding of health care is fundamental to such discussions and is considered in the next section.

The necessity for government involvement in the financing of health care

Chapter 1 briefly introduced the nature of the market mechanism and its operation in securing an efficient allocation of resources. However, in order for the market mechanism to deliver Pareto-efficiency, a number of conditions need to exist:
(1) Perfect competition:
  - a large number of consumers and suppliers, so that no one consumer or supplier can collude to exert excessive influence within the market;
  - product or service homogeneity, so that no one product or service can be distinguished from (and possibly have an advantage over) another;
  - complete freedom of entry into the market and exit from it, so that there are no constraints on new suppliers joining the market or existing suppliers leaving.
(2) Perfect knowledge on the part of consumers, so that consumers are fully aware of the characteristics of the product and/or service being provided,

know whether they want it, know how much they want, know when they want it and where they can get it.

(3) A certain world, where consumers can choose and plan when and where they will engage in transactions.

(4) Absence of externalities, which arise when the activities of one consumer and/or supplier affect the outcome of the activities of another agent and are not covered by the market mechanism.

In the real world, perfect competition does not exist. Markets are characterised by monopolistic tendencies and other structures that allow individual suppliers to exercise considerable control over the price to be charged or the amount to be produced. Even if perfect competition did exist, there are certain types of goods that either would not be provided at all or would be provided inadequately or in insufficient quantity by private firms. The demand side of the market mechanism is characterised by a desire for a commodity plus an ability to pay for it. For many products this may be perfectly realistic but for a range of others, it may not be. The characteristics of 'public goods' mean that such commodities are provided by central or local government (e.g. defence, street lighting) or not at all. In addition, governments intervene to finance and provide 'merit' goods, that is, goods and services that are higher on society's preference listing than on an aggregation of individuals' preference listings, alongside private suppliers. Examples of these are to be found in the provision of education, transport and health care. It is inconceivable that many people would be prepared to directly pay for the provision of speed cameras or traffic-calming schemes, designed to reduce the number of accidents, and it is left to government to provide such schemes.

Another problem associated with the operation of the market mechanism is the existence of what are called externalities. There are many examples of externalities in health care that require government intervention. In recent years, the dangers of passive smoking have been recognised and led to the introduction of smoking bans in public places, with New York, Italy and Ireland being prime examples. Such measures to counter the 'adverse effects' resulting from the activities of some members of society on others would not be possible if there were no government intervention in the operation of the market mechanism. Similarly, if there were no regulation and intervention on the 'supply side' to ensure that practitioners were qualified, the market would not prevent anyone from setting up as a practitioner, with potentially serious and even fatal consequences. While regulations and licensure do not necessarily guarantee that 'quacks' and 'one-offs' will not practice, the standards, skills and knowledge required for qualification go a long way in protecting the safety and interests of consumers, who are unlikely to be sufficiently informed to do so themselves.

Similarly, it is unrealistic to assume that consumers have, or can access, sufficient information relating to health care services (despite the wealth of information available from the Internet), to furnish themselves with the perfect knowledge required to make the decisions necessary when confronted by sickness and illness. Consumers of health care services, as in other areas, are therefore reliant on agents who act on their behalf – health care professionals. Agency arises in situations in which potential consumers recognise that they are not sufficiently well equipped to make rational, informed consumption decisions. They decide to rely on experts acting on their behalf so that they have a better chance of maximising utility. While politicians and policymakers have recognised the importance of involving patients in the decision-making processes and the role of the 'expert patient' has been developed, it is still the case that patients are generally ill-informed and that health care professionals are able to act as the more informed agent on behalf of patients, in relation to problem diagnoses, treatment availability and the effectiveness of interventions.

Other reasons that necessitate government involvement in the funding of health care services, as opposed to reliance on a private insurance-based system, arise due to the existence of adverse selection and moral hazard. Adverse selection occurs when people do not reveal the full extent of their health profile, and thereby their risk level, to the insurer. This may result in people at high risk paying lower premiums than their actual risk would indicate. As a consequence, insurers would inflate the premiums and some people may be left uninsured – those at low risk who do not bother to take up insurance as the premiums are too high and those at high risk who cannot afford the premiums.

Moral hazard arises when the attitudes and behaviours of people change once they are covered for the potential costs of treatment. They may choose to take less care of themselves and consume all health care services that they are entitled to, irrespective of whether they are needed or not. Chapter 1 made reference to the notion of 'flat of the curve' medicine,[1] which arises when the benefits generated from additional spending are unproductive and may only serve to fulfil the wants and desires of the 'insured' rather than any specific health care needs that they may have.

It is therefore apparent that there are powerful arguments in favour of government intervention in health care provision. What is also evident is that the market mechanism would not adequately deal with the supply of professionals. In theory, a market for health care professionals could exist, but there would be no system of qualification and regulation, and patients would have to choose between practitioners based on their own assessments of quality and price,[12] while there would be no curbs on overprovision of health care services, and, given the lack of knowledge and expertise among consumers of health care services, they would be utterly dependent on doctors and other health care professionals as their agents.

The role of health care professionals

The motivation of individuals who work within public services in general and within health care in particular has been widely discussed in the literature. Much of this concentrates on the extent to which such individuals are self-interested or altruistic.[13] However, most of the literature on organisational behaviour has made fairly simple assumptions concerning individual motivations and has concentrated on the extent to which individuals or groups of individuals with different motivational structures interact within organisations to affect organisational behaviour.

The economic theory of the firm provides three models to assess the behaviour of organisations. The first group of models is based on what is known as the traditional theory, which represent the firm as a single agent in pursuit of profit maximisation. The single firm is unable to exert any influence over the prices or levels of production, due to the fact that there are many other firms operating within the same market. Such models have very limited application in explaining the behaviour of organisations in general, yet alone those in health care services assume the existence of perfect competition in markets and bear no resemblance to the nature and complexity of the modern organisation.

The second group of models is based on the distinction between management and ownership and is known as 'managerial theories of the firm'.[14] These models also consider firms as single agents, but ones that pursue other goals not linked to profit maximisation, such as the maximisation of revenue. Managers will have different goals and objectives in relation to the performance of organisations than the owners of the organisation. For example, it was suggested that the short-term nature of managerial contracts within the NHS could, in some cases, result in decisions being made to protect their employment rather than other desirable, longer-term goals, such as staff or service development.[15]

The third group of models – multiple agent models, derived from behavioural theories of organisational behaviour – regards organisational behaviour as the product of multiple groups interacting within the organisation. Behavioural models[16] take cognisance of the complexities underlying organisations and describe the firm as a coalition of groups with conflicting interests. The firm is a 'satisficing' organisation rather than a maximising entity, which aims to achieve a number of objectives, such as the 'maximisation' of production levels, sales, market share and profit, but with equal emphasis on stability and survival. These behavioural models have been further developed to acknowledge the significance of relationships and interactions within the organisation and how behaviour is influenced through contracts and other forms of incentive structures.[17–19] Another type of model has been advocated as a logical variation on the behavioural model, which suggests that organisational motivation is the product of multiple actors, but with a dominant single actor mimicking the behaviour of the atomistic firm structure with a single overriding goal.[20]

Models of hospital behaviour have been drawn from the theoretical perspectives of organisational behaviour and the economic theories of the firm. Some have treated the hospital as a profit-maximising entity, in general assuming that clinicians are the primary decision-makers, while other models predict that other forms of maximisation exist which identify administrators as the decision-making unit.[21] Within the UK, managers and health care professionals have been identified as the principal actors within the NHS,[22,23] who coexist in a power coalition while harbouring different and potentially conflicting sets of interests. There was no consensus on whether either the managerial or the professional body was dominant but, within professionals, consultants were considered to be the dominant actors, over and above, say, nurses.[24] Much of the organisational change within the NHS during the 1980s and 1990s was an attempt to redefine the balance of power between doctors and managers, that is, to strengthen the role of management and to encourage participation by doctors in management, with the aim of shifting doctors' orientation and behaviour to be more like that of managers, thus strengthening the management's objective function of the NHS organisation.

However, such attempts were not without their casualties. A dramatic example of conflict between managers and medical staff took place in South Wales in 1995. An NHS Trust ran into serious financial difficulties, partly because medical staff were able to resist the implementation of a plan to make them redundant and to transfer others to another Trust when the service they were providing was to be transferred. In the battle that ensued – including a vote of no confidence in the Chairman of the Trust Board and the Chief Executive of the hospital passed by the medical staff – the Chairman and the Chief Executive of the Trust were replaced and the affair became the subject of an investigation by the Welsh Affairs Select Committee and Public Accounts Committee of the House of Commons.

More recent work has been undertaken to assess the extent to which the desire to strengthen the role of management and the participation of professionals in management had become apparent in reality and to determine whether in fact there is a dominant power base underlying decision-making in NHS Trusts. A survey of 1500 consultants and mangers (as the major power sources) across 100 Trusts was undertaken over a 3-year period to assess what motivating factors lay behind their agendas and eventually the performance of their Trusts.[20] The findings were that consultants considered production goals to be more important than financial break-even targets, but within those goals, considered quality to be more important than service volume. While the break-even target was generally found to be the primary goal of managers, they proved to be a heterogeneous group with quality ranking as the main priority among those managers who were closest to service delivery. This was at odds with the apparent objective of Trusts, which both groups perceived as being the pursuit of financial targets, consistent with the formal, government-set requirements. The study concluded that the reforms of previous years had done nothing to reduce the power base of the hospital consultant and that the Trusts' primary objective was to maintain service quality.

But what of the primary care sector where the context is complicated by the existence of other factors and situations? While the literature has concentrated on hospitals and NHS Trusts, the same imperatives apply in terms of service quality and financial targets in primary care, but issues relating to equity, wider efficiency objectives and indeed ethical considerations also impinge significantly on the objectives and behaviour of primary care organisations. In addition, there are also the potential conflicts that arise from the different agendas, and objective functions that arise from the role of health care professionals as agents, especially in the context of primary care, with its dual functions of service commissioning and service provision.

Health care professionals as the agents of patients

The role of the health care professional as the agent of the patient is of particular relevance to the organisation of health care services.[12,25,26] The health care professional is in the unenviable position of wearing one hat as health care service provider and, at the same time, having to wear the hat of patient advisor. As providers they seek to diagnose, treat and care for the health care needs and problems faced by patients. As patients' agents, they aim to put themselves in the place of the patients and provide advice, based on their greater knowledge and expertise, to inform the patients, who can then address their health care needs. In other words, the objectives and goals of health care professionals should mirror those of their patients. This, of course, assumes close correspondence between the health care needs of patients as perceived by patients themselves and those as perceived by health care professionals.

Much energy and effort has gone into the assessment of needs of patients. Needs are categorised into those that are perceived and those that are not, by the patient or agent. The former relate to those that exist when an 'abnormality' is identified by the patient which can be dealt with in one, or a combination, of three ways:
(1) no action;
(2) use made of one of the informal agencies involved in health and social care, e.g. self-medication, informal carers;
(3) contact made with health care and social care services at the initial point of contact (i.e. 'expressed need').
Health care professionals may have a different perspective than that of patients, and it may be that the self-perceived needs of the patient are not acknowledged as being 'need' by health care professionals but rather as being 'neurosis'. Thus, because of this assessment by professionals, self-perceived needs would not necessarily be met with service provision.

The other category of needs, namely needs unperceived by the (potential) patient, would encompass conditions that are unrecognised by an individual, the family, carers or friends but that are potentially discoverable by practitioners and professionals on careful investigation of the total physical, mental and emotional well-being of the individual.[27] The problem is that they only become discoverable when patients make contact with the service providers, who then take on the responsibility of agents acting on their behalf. Such needs may warrant intervention (when it is thought that prevention, management or specific therapy would be of benefit) but would also include those situations where intervention to meet such needs may prove to be unwanted by the patient, e.g. a severe warning to change lifestyle behaviour and habits if serious coronary events are to be avoided.

For some people, the ability to identify or articulate their needs is extremely difficult, while for most lay people their limited knowledge does present a major constraint in equating needs with appropriate interventions and services. The problem is also compounded by the fact that in the case of health care, patients' reliance on professional advice may lead to potentially difficult and contentious situations. Suppliers of services are, potentially, in a very advantageous situation when needs have to be assessed, especially when the two functions (assessor and supplier) are contained within the same agency. Reference was made in Chapter 1 to the number of unnecessary treatments,[28] while the 'manufacture' of illnesses and their ongoing sustenance has also been highlighted.

> First described in 1953 in the US, whiplash rapidly achieved notoriety ...within ten years it had become a subject heading in the Cumulated Index Medicus...and quickly became a worldwide epidemic and a multibillion-dollar industry...with a current estimate of £3.1 billion in UK.[29]

This sort of example raises the obvious question of whether service provision is patient-led, with health care professionals acting as agents of patients, or whether the supply of such services is driven by professional, organisational, political and economic interests. Supply-induced demand has been defined as 'the extent to which a doctor provides or recommends the provision of medical services that differ from what the patient would choose if he or she had available the same information and knowledge as the physician'.[30] The question as to whether need exists may not be relevant,[26] but it is important to realise that there may not be a coincidence between the views of patients and those of the professionals regarding needs. The perceptions of GPs, nurses and patients may all differ. For example, the relationship between patient and doctor has been portrayed in an amusing, but probably reasonably accurate, way:[31]

> At the heart of clinical practice is the doctor–patient relationship. In principle this is a principal–agent relationship in which the patient is principal and the doctor the agent. If a doctor is acting as the perfect agent of his patient, their respective roles would be that the DOCTOR is there to give the PATIENT all the information the PATIENT needs in order that the PATIENT can make a decision, and the DOCTOR should

implement that decision once the PATIENT has made it. If that does not sound quite the way it usually is, try reversing the roles of DOCTOR and PATIENT, so that the relationship now gets described as the PATIENT being there to give the DOCTOR all the information the DOCTOR needs in order that the DOCTOR can make a decision, and the PATIENT should then implement that decision once the DOCTOR has made it.

The question as to who should assess the needs of patients and how they should be responded to cannot be answered on empirical grounds alone. The question is ultimately both subjective and political and goes to the very heart of the theories of moral justice. What can help in practice is for managers and professionals to be clear about their own particular values and ideas surrounding the notions of justice and equality but also to recognise that other views, in particular those of the patient, need to be borne in mind.

The relationship between health care needs and individual desires

It may be that health care needs do not correspond totally to the desires of individuals with regard to their health – partly because of some needs being identified by someone other than the patient and partly because some things that we need might not necessarily be wanted and vice versa. In addition, desires and needs are not independent of the level of supply available, and may be based upon knowledge and awareness of the existence of certain facilities. Such facilities and services have often been provided for elderly people and others requiring care provision by agents on the basis of factors other than their needs or wants. The case of Mrs Green has been used to demonstrate how the perceived needs of the service recipient did not correspond with the assessment of needs undertaken by the health and social services authorities. Mrs Green's desire (and need?) was for her garden to be kept tidy, but the 'official assessment' determined that she needed community nursing and occupational health inputs and attendance at a local day care centre.[32]

The proportion of an individual's needs that are actually met by care services is subject to debate, but even if the proportion were approaching 100% for one person, this is unlikely to be regarded as equitable or fair, if for other people the proportion was much lower. In such a situation inequities and inequalities are possibly being compounded rather than reduced. In addition, should those whose own actions create a need for care services (e.g. heavy smokers or drug abusers) be treated differently from those who have similar needs through no 'fault' of their own? The notions of 'comparative need' and 'relative need' thus have to be brought into consideration, and this is where the professionals have an important role to play, subject to the proviso mentioned above, that they should be prepared to make explicit their

Box 2.1 New Figures Reveal Hidden Epidemic of Self-harm

Britain is facing a spiralling epidemic of self-harm, shocking new figures indicate. More than 170,000 people a year – most of them teenagers and young adults – seek hospital treatment after deliberately hurting themselves in apparent expressions of despair, research has found.

Source: Maxine Frith, Social Affairs Correspondent (*The Independent* 27 July 2004). *http://news.independent.co.uk/uk/health_medical/story.jsp?story = 545105* (accessed 30 December 2004)

own values and ideas of justice and equity and recognise that other views are also important.

In addition, it is highly likely that many of the demands placed on health care services by consumers are also unnecessary, based not on specific health care needs but on other life problems, or arising out of health-damaging behaviour, which people believe that the health care system can fix. It has been reported that more than 50% of the population of England is currently overweight or obese, and it is known that obesity reduces life expectancy by 9 years on average. There was a 25% increase in the number of overweight or obese children between 1995 and 2002. In contrast, just 40% of men and 26% of women take enough exercise – defined as 30 min of moderately intense physical activity on five or more occasions per week.[33] Furthermore, the ever-increasing incidence and prevalence of substance abuse and self-harm add to the pressures confronting the health service, as highlighted in Box 2.1.

In addition, there are people who feel ill and present to the health care system, but in whom there is no underlying pathology or disease.[34] This phenomenon has been attributed to medically unexplained physical symptoms (MUPS) or hypochondriasis.[35] The extent of such disorders is not insignificant, with about 50% of people attending general medicine outpatients estimated to have MUPS.[35] Low back pain, for example, has been referred to as a twentieth-century disaster,[36] in that over the past 20 years or so there has emerged an 'epidemic of chronic disability attributed to non-specific low back pain and an increase in associated sick certification and disability and incapacity benefits, for which there is no good medical explanation and which appears to be largely a social phenomenon'.[37] In more recent times, low back pain may have become 'less sexy' and stress and other minor psychological problems have emerged as the 'disease' that requires a psychosocial, as well as medical, diagnostic and treatment regimen.[38]

The existence of such phenomena has called into question the underlying models of illness. It has been argued that most models of illness assume a causal relation between disease and illness and that removal or attenuation of the disease will result in a return to health, since health is the absence of disease.[39] It has been suggested that many of the stresses and strains witnessed in health care and illness-related benefit systems can be attributed to the emphasis on the biomedical model, and that greater emphasis should be placed on the biopsychosocial model, which assumes that disease is only one of the factors contributing to illness and illness behaviour, in order to facilitate improvement in delivery of health care and reduce incapacity to work.[39]

Therefore, in considering the level of funding required and the approaches and options available and appropriate to finance the provision of health care services, there are a wide variety of stakeholders and interest groups, whose views and perspectives need to be taken into account. In no particular order of priority they include patients and their representatives, professionals and their respective professional bodies, managers, policymakers and politicians, ethicists, the pharmaceutical industry and other providers of health equipment, insurance companies involved in health care, academic researchers and, not least, the taxpaying public. All of these groups have different goals and agendas in relation to the level of health care funding and how it is organised, and therefore it is worth prefacing the next section by emphasising that there is no single correct system for organising the funding of health care in a country and that there are pros and cons associated with each approach.

Funding health care services

The Wanless Report, published in 2002, highlighted that in order to secure an improvement in the quality of the services provided in the UK, expenditure on health care services would have to increase towards 12% of gross domestic product (GDP) – an increase from the current £68 billion to well over £150 billion (2002/03 prices) on the best estimates and over £180 billion when less favourable estimates are used.[10] However, as highlighted in Chapter 1, the resources available for health services (public or private) are finite and the health care dilemma forces governments and decision-makers to make choices, which at times are extremely difficult. The ever-increasing demand for health care services against a background of limited resources – emphasised by current shortages among doctors – that is likely to be exacerbated during the foreseeable future as fewer people apply for places in medical schools has been addressed by a number of broad policy options, with varying degrees of success. These are briefly outlined below.

Increase efficiency

This option covers a whole variety of themes ranging from reducing the costs of catering or domestic services (through competitive tendering) to reducing the unit costs of treating patients through, for example, a move from inpatient surgery to day case surgery. The overall aim is the same, to get the health care services to deliver more care for the same amount of money. Broadly speaking, the recent reforms to the NHS in the UK have been primarily concerned with promoting greater efficiency in service delivery. However, as demonstrated in Chapter 1 the drive for greater efficiency may result in equity in health having to be compromised.

Limit service range

The term prioritisation or its negative version, rationalisation, have become part of everyday usage within health care systems in recent years. As a process, it is an 'elaborate and intricate issue'[40] and also highly emotive.

For example, the funding of the so-called 'lifestyle drug' Viagra became one of the major elements in debates surrounding the rationing of health care interventions. The government argued that the mechanisms of funding this type of intervention might even threaten the financial sustainability of current health systems, with the Secretary of State for Health making the case that, with regard to clinical need, impotence could not be regarded as a priority for any additional NHS expenditure compared with cancer, heart disease and mental health since, while it may result in psychological distress, it was not life-threatening or causing physical pain.[41]

Another example of the issues revolving around establishing priorities was found in the case of child B, a ten-year-old girl suffering from acute myeloid leukaemia. After a bone marrow transplant, the disease appeared to have been cured but the leukaemia returned and clinicians told the girl's father that she had only a few weeks to live. He contacted a private practitioner who was willing to treat child B with a new treatment that would cost £75 000. The HA refused to fund the treatment or provide a second bone marrow transplant since expert opinion was that the chances of success were extremely slim. A high-profile legal battle ensued and eventually the Court of Appeal found in favour of the HA. An anonymous benefactor provided the funds for the treatment and the girl survived for another year before a further relapse led to her death. Although this particular example achieved national media attention, priority-setting decisions involving ethical and other cost-effective considerations are at the heart of policies and local decision-making on an everyday basis.

The establishment of NICE sought to address the problems associated with 'postcode prescribing', where services and treatments were available in one area but not in a neighbouring location. Before NICE the process of limiting the range of services made available had been ad hoc and not without considerable controversy, as evidenced in the two examples above, but the extent to which NICE has succeeded has yet to be proved.[42]

Additional funding

The option favoured by most NHS staff and, according to opinion polls, by a large proportion of the general public would be to increase the level of funds going into the existing NHS. This could be done in a number of ways, such as levying charges, increasing taxation proceeds or shifting resources from other parts of the public sector. What is not evident, however, is the extent to which additional resources will translate into additional health benefits, and to whom they would accrue. Additional resources may prove to be very welcome but if they are channelled into inappropriate areas, the result may be greater inefficiency and wider inequalities. The contrasting situations in terms of expenditure and indicators of health status from the USA and Japan were highlighted in Chapter 1, while the comparison between the NHS and Kaiser Permanente[11] also challenge such a view. The question is whether additional resources to improve job prospects and reduce poverty, for example, would result in greater health care benefits than would be gained from additional expenditure on health care facilities and treatments.

Alternative financing structure

A fourth alternative would be to completely restructure the method of organising and funding health services. In the UK, this could involve the deployment of some form of health insurance system. For example, 500 hospital consultants issued a call for the radical reform of the NHS to put power into patients' hands, by taking out a full-page advertisement in *The Times* on 25 February 2004. The group, entitled Doctors for Reform, stated their commitment to the NHS ideals of equitable and universal health care but believed that this could be better achieved by other methods of financing. Professor Karol Sikora, an oncologist and one of the founder members of the group, said:

> The NHS as we know it has had its day. You can fiddle about with it and patch it up, but with an ageing population and high-tech health care, something has to give. Everything else we need today we can get very easily: air travel, holidays, cars. Why can't we get health care that easily? The form of funding is the key. To change it is a radical step. Politicians are very nervous. But we have to do it if we want a system that is focused on the patient and open to innovative ideas.[43]

However, there is no guarantee that changes in the financing structures will generate improvement in performance. While there is some evidence of excess demand for health care services and insufficient supply of health care resources in the UK compared to other countries – for example, it was shown that UK had 50% of the number of beds per 1000 population compared to France in 2000[44] – many of the problems that face the NHS in the UK and health systems in other countries are not primarily a function of their funding arrangements. They are in fact multifactorial, resulting from factors such as external cost pressures on pharmaceuticals and other medical equipment and devices, growing demands from an expanding and increasingly articulate and informed population, and pressures on the supply of human resources resulting from demographic changes and legislation relating to working conditions.

The World Health Organization (WHO) produced a report in 2000 that sought to establish criteria to assess the performance of health care systems across the world. The five goals against which each health care system was to be judged were maximisation of population health, reducing inequalities in the health of populations, maximising responsiveness, reducing inequalities in responsiveness and financing health care in a fair manner.[45] However, while the intention was generally sound and there was considerable analysis to support the work, the quality of the underlying database was of dubious quality, with an excessive reliance on estimates.[46]

What is evident is that it is extremely difficult to identify which health systems are the most efficient[46,47] and which secure the greatest 'benefit per buck' for its residents.

Reduce demand for health services

A key policy plank of most governments would be to try and reduce the demand for health services by preventing people from getting ill in the first place. It has been estimated that preventable illness constitutes approximately 70% of the burden of illness and the associated costs[48] and therefore the incentives to utilise health promotion and preventive measures for such a purpose are obviously attractive.

However, there are two basic issues at stake: firstly, is there evidence that prevention and health promotion reduce health care costs; and secondly, whether any health care programme or intervention should be assessed in relation to its impact on financial budgets? In response to the first it is surely the prime objective of any health care intervention or programme to improve the health of the particular patients or community, which as a result may secure reductions in costs to the health service and patients and communities. The same principle should apply to any consideration of prevention and health promotion, and the more appropriate question is whether additional resources spent on prevention or health promotion would generate greater health benefits than if those resources had been used elsewhere?

The second issue has grown in importance recently as purchasers have to operate within constrained budgets. The publication of guidance and guidelines, even when based on quality evidence, can have a profound impact on available resources. For example, it was argued that implementation of the guidance on statins in patients at high risk of coronary heart disease could potentially cost a single HA in the UK roughly 20% of its annual drug budget.[49] While health economic evaluation can be utilised in decisions relating to the prioritisation of services, it is not sufficient to predict whether they are affordable within available budgets. It is becoming usual for budget impact assessment to be included alongside economic evaluations when evidence is submitted to agencies deciding on formulary inclusion or reimbursement. More attention is devoted to this process in Chapter 6.

The plethora of different forms of health care systems around the world, with their different forms of financing and organising the delivery of health care services, seems to imply that there is no single, unique or right way of doing things. It could also mean that different systems have evolved to suit different societies with different cultures, ideas and notions of medicine, the citizen's right to care and so on. What is evident, however, is that systems are continually changing and evolving. So how much should be spent on health and health care? Who should decide?

Expenditure on health care services

As shown in Figure 2.1, there is considerable variation between countries in the levels of health care expenditure. However, it does not necessarily mean that countries at the top of the chart, with a greater share of their GDP allocated to health, have the best returns from such expenditure and those at the bottom have the worst, as evidenced by the comparison made between the situations in Japan and the USA.

As can be seen from Figure 2.1, there is a distinction made between public sector and private sector health care expenditure, but this, in many senses, is an oversimplification. For example, within the UK, certain medication is available over the counter at the local pharmacist, but only some people are entitled to 'free' treatments as prescribed by their GP. The same distinctions apply to aspects of dental care, ophthalmic services, etc., where some sections of the population receive the services without having to pay directly, while

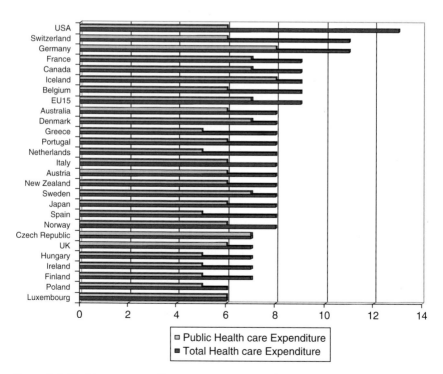

Figure 2.1 Health care expenditure as a percentage of GDP in OECD countries.

others have to pay the full amount. Distinctions and differences also apply in other countries, with some people entitled to full reimbursement on any costs incurred in treatments, while others are only entitled to a percentage of the full amount.

Different approaches to financing

There are in essence four basic alternative methods of financing care services:
(1) Direct payment by users
(2) Private health insurance
(3) Social or state insurance
(4) Direct tax
All health care systems are essentially pluralistic with respect to financing (and delivery), with tendencies towards one method rather than another. For example, in the USA the health care economy is dominated by private health insurance but with a significant proportion of government-funded care, while in Switzerland, 25% of total health expenditure comes from social insurance, 33% from direct payments and 40% from general taxes.

In Chapter 1, consideration was given to the concept of health as distinguished from health care, and the idea propounded that by spending more on factors external to the health care system less would be required by the health care system. Obviously this question is addressed to the notion of state funding rather than any individual decision to purchase more health and social care. Four practical approaches have been suggested to the problem of determining the level of state funding of health and social care.[50] They are:
(1) Incremental funding
(2) Incremental funding linked to affordability
(3) International comparisons
(4) Democratic decision

Incremental funding
This approach involves looking at current levels of expenditure and then making some changes at the margin to produce a new budget for the next year. However, with this approach no account is taken of the allocation of funds within the system; demographic changes are not considered; medical advances and technological changes are ignored; health policy developments are not taken into consideration; and any fundamental underfunding of the system is not dealt with.

Incremental funding linked to affordability
Such an approach ties increases in health care expenditure to increases in the wealth of the nation – GDP. Hence, one would expect public expenditure on health and social care to be a constant percentage of GDP.

However, there are two major problems with this approach. Firstly, what happens when GDP is falling or only rising marginally? There is evidence to suggest that demand for health care resources increases during recessionary periods, which suggests that the relationship between health expenditure and GDP is inverse. Should this be reflected in the way health expenditure levels are tied to GDP or should there be a minimum baseline growth in health expenditure, which negates the rationale for a GDP linkage?

The second criticism relates to the political implications for governments in seeking to tie health care expenditure to GDP growth. It is highly unlikely that any government would willingly surrender their control of a proportion of public spending to a formula that dictated spending levels. Furthermore, there may well be pressure to encourage private health expenditure and reduce the burden on the public purse, as well as from private sector providers themselves, to increase 'market share', to maintain parity with GDP. The distributive effects of such a policy would in all probability exacerbate inequalities in health care as private health care would not be attainable for the low paid, high risk and uninsurable.

International comparisons

This is an oft-quoted statistic but one which is very unreliable as an indicator. Not only is it difficult to collect comparable data but interpreting the data and drawing conclusions from such data are highly susceptible to criticisms (e.g. cultural factors, differences in definitions, differences in demographic and epidemiological patterns). Other issues arise due to the nature of comparisons made. For example, currency fluctuations can result in major changes in comparisons without any actual change in expenditure. An alternative approach has been the use of purchasing power parities, which relate to the cost of health care to the economy as a whole, having made allowance for differences in the level of general prices between countries. However, differences in the price of health care products and services are not necessarily accounted for, and so another approach has been to employ health care–specific purchasing power parities. The reliability of these data and the complexities and differences between health care systems means that extreme caution should be taken in using international comparisons in seeking to establish the appropriate level of spending on health care.

Democratic decision

The issue surrounding levels of health care expenditure is essentially a normative one, based on value judgements. Within democracies the voting system, in theory at least, is the means by which difficult issues involving value judgements can be resolved. However, in reality this is often not the case. A number of government policies are not necessarily contained within election manifestos and therefore do not appear before the electorate for their consideration and approval. In addition the question of who votes is very important. A number of groups within society are disenfranchised, some of whom are heavy users of resources in health and social care, while others are unable to vote because of disability, infirmity, etc.

Opinion polls are alternative ways of acquiring the views of society but these suffer from methodological problems, and while there are some examples of community-wide surveys and ballots relating to the issue of funding health and social care, there is no evidence to date of them penetrating into political agendas.

The inadequacies of outcome measures also compound the problems in seeking to reach a consensus as to what level of funding is appropriate, and one is left with the inevitable conclusion that if democracy is to have any say in the arguments, it hinges on the amount of imperfection that one is prepared to tolerate in the information available and in the methodologies used to acquire the views of the community.

The question as to how much should actually be spent on health care services was addressed at a conference following publication of the Wanless Report.[10] It is worth quoting the conclusion reached by the editors of the publication resulting from the conference:

> As already alluded to, it is not possible to reduce a review of future spending to a technical exercise (albeit a very complicated one) (i.e the Wanless review). There are questions of value (particularly in a non-marketed service such as the NHS) which are best addressed not by economists, politicians or Treasury policy wonks, but by society more generally. There are also prior questions about the sort of NHS we want – the 'vision' – and what we are prepared to sacrifice in order to achieve it. No amount of modelling, no matter how sophisticated, will help answer such vital questions – rather, they require consideration by those to whom the NHS is ultimately accountable: the public and patients.[51]

References

1 Mitton C, Donaldson C. *Priority setting toolkit: a guide to the use of economics in healthcare decision making.* London: BMJ Books, 2004.
2 Sussex J. *The economics of the private finance initiative in the NHS.* London: Office of Health Economics, 2001.
3 Pollock AM, Shaoul J, Vickers N. Private finance and "value for money" in NHS hospitals: a policy in search of a rationale? *BMJ* 2002; 324: 1205–209.
4 Department of Health. *Working for patients.* London: HMSO, 1989.
5 Baggott R. *Health and health care in Britain.* London: Macmillan, 1998.
6 Le Grand J. Competition, cooperation or control? Tales from the British Health Service. *Health Affairs* 1999; 18: 27–39.
7 Le Grand J. Further tales from the British Health Service. *Health Affairs* 2002; 21: 116–28.
8 Department of Health. *The new NHS: modern, dependable.* London: HMSO, 1997.
9 Shifrin T. NHS faces 'retirement timebomb'. *The Guardian* 23 August 2004. *http://www.guardian.co.uk/uk_news/story/0%2C3604%2C1289121%2C00.html* (accessed 26 September 2004)

10 Wanless D. *Securing our future health: taking a long-term view.* London: HM Treasury, 2002. *http://www.hm-treasury.gov.uk./Consultations_and_Legislation/wanless/consult_wanless_final.cfm* (accessed 17 October 2004)

11 Feachem RGA, Sekhri NK, White KL. Getting more for their dollar: a comparison of the NHS with California's Kaiser Permanente. *BMJ* 2002; 324: 135–43.

12 Donaldson C, Gerard K. *Economics of health care financing: the visible hand.* Basingstoke: Macmillan, 1993.

13 Le Grand J. *Motivation, agency and public policy: of knight and knaves, pawns and queens.* Oxford: Oxford University Press, 2003.

14 Baumol WJ. *Business behavior value and growth.* New York: Macmillan, 1959.

15 Ferlie E. Increasing top management turnover: is it true and does it matter? *J Health Services Res Policy* 1997; 2: 1–2.

16 Cyert RM, March JG. *A behavioural theory of the firm.* New Jersey: Prentice-Hall, 1963.

17 Williamson OE. Transaction cost economics: the governance of contractual relations. *J Law Econ* 1979; 22: 233–62.

18 Deitrich M. *Transaction cost economics and beyond: towards a new theory of the firm.* London: Routledge, 1994.

19 Putterman L. *The economic nature of the firm: a reader.* New York: Cambridge University Press, 1986.

20 Crilly T, Le Grand J. The motivation and behaviour of hospital trusts. *Soc Sci Med* 2004; 58: 1809–23.

21 McGuire A. The theory of the hospital: a review of the models. *Soc Sci Med* 1985; 20(11): 1177–85.

22 Ferlie E, Ashburner L, Fitzgerald L *et al. The new public management in action.* Oxford: Oxford University Press, 1996.

23 Harrison S, Pollitt C. *Controlling health professionals: the future of work and organisation in the NHS.* Buckingham: Open University Press, 1994.

24 Walby S, Greenwell J, Mackay L *et al. Medicine and nursing: professions in changing health service.* London: Sage, 1994.

25 Mooney G. *Economics, medicine and health care.* London: Harvester Wheatsheaf, 1992.

26 Mooney G. *Key issues in health economics.* Hemel Hempstead: Harvester Wheatsheaf, 1994.

27 Alderson M. *An introduction to epidemiology.* Basingstoke: Macmillan, 1993.

28 Borowitz M, Sheldon T. Controlling health care: from economic interventions to micro-clinical regulation. *Health Econ* 1993; 2: 201–204.

29 Mallenson A. *Whiplash and other useful illnesses.* Montreal: McGill-Queen's University Press, 2002.

30 Rice TH. The impact of changing medicare reimbursement rates on physician-induced demand. *Med Care* 1983; 21: 803–15.

31 Williams A. Ethics, clinical freedom and the doctors' role, in Culyer AJ, Maynard A, Posnett J (eds). *Competition in health care: reforming the NHS.* Basingstoke: Macmillan, 1990.

32 Palfrey C, Thomas P, Phillips CJ. *Effective healthcare management: an evaluative approach.* Oxford: Blackwell, 2004.

33 Wanless D. *Securing good health for the whole population.* London: HM Treasury, 2004. *http://www.hm-treasury.gov.uk./media/E43/27/Wanless04_summary.pdf* (accessed 12 January 2004)

34 Carson AJ, Ringbauer B, Stone J *et al.* Do medically unexplained symptoms matter? A prospective cohort study of 300 new referrals to neurology outpatient clinics. *J Neurol Neurosurg Psychiatry* 2000; 68: 207–10.

35 Muir Gray JA. *Evidence-based healthcare.* Edinburgh: Churchill Livingstone, 1997.

36 Waddell G. *The back pain revolution.* Edinburgh: Churchill Livingstone, 1998.

37 Waddell G, Aylward M, Sawney P. *Back pain, incapacity for work and social security benefits: an international literature review and analysis.* London: Royal Society of Medicine Press, 2002.

38 Aylward M. Personal communication, 2004.

39 Wade DT, Halligan PW. Do biodmedical models of illness make for good healthcare systems? *BMJ* 2004; 329: 1398–401.

40 Coast J, Donovan J. Conflict, complexity and confusion: the context for priority setting, in Coast J, Donovan J, Frankel S (eds). *Priority setting: the health care debate.* London: Wiley and Sons, 1996.

41 Gilbert D, Walley T, New B. Lifestyle medicines. *BMJ,* 2000; 321: 1341–44.

42 Dent THS, Sadler M. From guidance to practice: why NICE is not enough. *BMJ,* 2002; 324: 842–45.

43 Hawkes N. Doctors want all ill patients to buy insurance. *The Times* 25 February 2004.

44 Jacobzone S. Resource and service implications of short waiting time: the French experience, in Appleby J, Devlin N, Dawson D (eds). *How much should we spend on the NHS?* London: Office of Health Economics, 2004.

45 WHO report 2000. *http://www.who.int/whr/2000/en/whr00_en.pdf* (accessed 16 January 2005)

46 Williams A. Science or marketing at WHO? A commentary on 'World Health 2000'. *Health Econ* 2001; 10: 93–100.

47 McPake B, Kumaranayake L, Normand C. *Health economics: an international perspective.* London: Routledge, 2002.

48 Fries JF, Koop CE, Beadle CE *et al.* Reducing health care costs by reducing the need and demand for medical services. *N Engl J Med* 1993; 329(5): 321–25.

49 Freemantle N, Barbour R, Johnson R *et al.* The use of statins: a case of misleading priorities. *BMJ* 1997; 315: 826–28.

50 Appleby J. *Financing health care in the 1990s.* Milton Keynes: Open University Press, 1992.

51 Appleby J, Devlin N, Dawson D. *How much should we spend on the NHS? Issues and challenges arising from the Wanless Review of future health care spending.* London: Office of Health Economics, 2004.

CHAPTER 3
The costs of health care

The aim of this chapter is to explore the notion of cost in health economics. The economist's notion of cost has already been described in Chapter 1, where the concept of *opportunity cost* was introduced. This concept is fundamental within economics. Because resources are scarce, choices have to be made between competing claims on the resources and, in making such choices, sacrifices and costs are incurred. The nature of choices, which have to be constantly made by individuals, professionals, organisations, governments and societies, is often complex with many other factors needing to be brought into the decision-making process.

What is cost?

It is important to stress at the outset that cost, in economic terms, is not only concerned with the financial imperatives. It has often been stated, incorrectly, that health economics is about saving money and reducing expenditure. In that case, health economists would not be assessing interventions and treatments that prolong life, or those that seek to prevent death, in terms of their relative cost-effectiveness, as they would be only concerned with spending less and focusing on programmes and policies that contributed to achieving an improvement in financial budgets rather than an improvement in the health of patients. In purely monetary terms, the cheapest patient is a dead patient!

The cost of using a resource in a particular service or treatment is, therefore, not (necessarily) the price that is paid for that resource but the benefit foregone (the opportunity lost) by not choosing the alternative. Successive UK governments, and those established since devolution, have placed considerable emphasis on the number of people on waiting lists and the length of time they have to wait to receive hospital treatment as an indicator of the relative success of the NHS. However, what is probably more important are the opportunity losses incurred by people, and by society, who await further treatment. There have been many examples of people who have died while waiting for cardiac treatment, while for others, the downward spiral into greater disability and dependency brings additional costs for themselves, their families and indeed for the health service and other agencies.

Initially, it is worth seeking to clarify some misconceptions relating to how economists arrive at the cost of services or interventions. Efforts to determine the cost of services and programmes from the perspective of a health economist are likely to differ from those employed by an accountant. For example, in costing a long-stay mental health facility, it was found that the staff spent most of their time caring for a small number of patients with the most serious problems, with very little direct support provided for the majority of patients. The actual use of staff resources and differences in the cost of provision of services between patients with serious problems and others would not have been identified if costs were calculated from accounting data alone.[1] Information recorded for accounting purposes would have identified the number of staff involved in the provision of care at the facility, the equipment, materials and drugs used and an allocation for overheads. This would then have been divided by the number of patients to provide the unit cost of care – that is the cost per patient – at the facility. However, from other information it is evident that such an approach does not adequately represent the actual cost profile of providing care for these patients. It is important to recognise that issues relating to economies of scale – where, for example, the underutilisation of a magnetic resonance imaging (MRI) scanner would result in a cost per procedure greater than if it were operating to full capacity – are taken into account. Similarly, it is important to be aware of cultural, organisational and specific patient characteristics that can lead to cost differentials – for example, differences between hospitals in relation to their policies on the admission and discharge of patients.

The process of costing health care services

There are basically three stages involved in the process of costing health care services and interventions[2]: (1) identification of costs (see Box 3.1); (2) measurement of identified costs; and (3) their translation into a monetary

---

Box 3.1 Types of Cost

Direct costs	These relate to the use of resources directly as a result of the treatment and health care process. They include drug acquisition costs, cost of nursing, medical and other staff time involved in delivering care and administering the procedures, costs of materials and equipment used in service provision, allocation of organisational overheads to the particular service PLUS costs to other organisations involved in the process AND to patients, in terms of time costs, transport costs and out-of-pocket expenses.

Continued

Box 3.1 Types of Cost—*Continued*

Indirect costs/productivity costs	These relate to 'losses' to society incurred as a result of the impact of disease, illness and treatments in preventing people from engaging in normal daily activities, such as work, domestic responsibilities and social and leisure engagements.
Intangibles	These relate to the distress, suffering, anxiety and impact on quality of life (QOL) resulting from illness and poor health and their treatments.

---

amount, bearing in mind that money may not always be the most representative indicator of opportunity cost.

Identification of costs

Identification of costs involves the listing of the likely resource effects of providing the service or intervention as comprehensively as possible (discussed in more detail in Chapter 5). Although this depends on the perspective being considered, it is possible to consider the costs of service provision from the perspective of the GP practice, or clinical directorate at one end of a spectrum to that of society at the other end.

Firstly, there are the direct costs, which can be subdivided into the direct health care costs, costs to other agencies resulting from health care provision and direct costs to patients and their families. These result from the time patients allocate to the receipt of health care services, the costs incurred in having to travel to and from health care facilities and other expenses, such as over-the-counter medication, purchasing equipment and aids to ease the burden of their conditions. In addition, it includes the time individuals devote to caring for relatives and friends, in conjunction with, or in place of, the formal care agencies.

Secondly, there are the indirect costs or productivity costs associated with health care. These occur outside the health care sector and relate to losses of production, due to absenteeism and reduced productivity, plus those incurred through the informal care process – as a result of a carer either giving up paid employment or sacrificing leisure time to provide care, which would otherwise have been provided by formal care agencies. In terms of work losses, this is called 'productivity costs'[3] – which refer to 'the costs associated with lost or impaired ability to work or to engage in leisure activities due to morbidity and lost economic productivity due to death'.[4]

Although the intangibles cause the biggest headache in terms of measurement and valuation, in essence they provide the biggest distinction between health care and other commodities. These are the things thatcan be identified by their very nature but have to be experienced to be measured and valued. A consultant in intensive care once told a conference audience that one of the most poignant moments of his career occurred in a trial to assess whether recovery in intensive care settings was improved if the patient was sedated or awake. One lady, when asked what the major benefit of being awake was, quietly but firmly informed him, 'being able to hold and feel my daughter's hand!' The impact of health problems on the QOL of patients, their families and communities is impossible to be contained within any financial statement. For example, Box 3.2 highlights some of the 'QOL costs' associated with a condition called atopic eczema.

The issues highlighted in Box 3.2 demonstrate that the importance of identifying as many of the costs as possible in the development of a cost profile cannot be overemphasised. Even though it may not be possible to measure and value all costs, it is essential that all costs associated with the programme be identified so that decision-makers are fully aware of *all* of the resource implications. In other words, the difficulties of quantification and valuation should not preclude the existence of all costs from the 'balance sheet' of costs and benefits to be considered by the decision-maker. The opportunity cost of not sensing the presence of the daughter's hand cannot be ignored.

While it may be desirable to identify all costs, in practice some are likely to be trivial and not worth collecting, or the costs involved may be excessive in

---

Box 3.2 The Quality-of-Life Impact of Atopic Eczema

Atopic eczema is a condition that has major impact on quality of life. The stress related to the care of a child with moderate or severe atopic eczema has been shown to be significantly greater than that of the care of children with insulin-dependent diabetes. Quality-of-life studies with patients and their families have highlighted considerable physical and psychological morbidity. For example, severe itching has resulted in sleep disturbance, with the consequential effects on siblings and parents, while engaging in normal childhood activities, hobbies and interests are often 'out-of-bounds' for children with atopic eczema. Many children have reported feeling 'different', embarrassed, isolated and subjected to teasing and bullying, which also leads to a general lack of confidence and 'school-phobia'. In addition, educational performance may also be affected as a result of the loss of schooling due to sleeplessness, side-effects of medication and loss of concentration caused by itching, which can have long-term consequences for patients. The impact of the condition on the work loss of parents is also highly significant, as they take time off work to visit health care professionals with their children. In addition, parents may have to reduce their working times or give up work altogether, while others may not even start employment.

Source: Phillips.[5]

relation to the benefits derived from such information. Evidence relating to costs is unlikely to be present at one single source, and information may have to be collected from databases, administrative records, case records and clinical trials, systematic reviews and observational studies or from staff in finance departments who may be rather unwilling to release what they regard as sensitive or confidential information. The quality of such evidence is variable and it is essential that the validity of assumptions and the impact of changes in costs be assessed in a sensitivity analysis when an economic evaluation is being undertaken.

Measurement of costs

Measurement of costs refers to the quantification of the resources used in providing the particular service – units of service. In deciding which costs to measure, it is usual to isolate those that are important and whose exclusion would bias the overall cost profile of the service or intervention. For those remaining, an assessment is made of the additional value added to the cost profile relative to the extra cost of collecting. Anything that is expensive to collect but whose inclusion is unlikely to influence the overall result need not be measured.

Costs are initially measured in relevant physical units such as hours of staff time, quantity of medication, equipment usage and number of patients being treated. In studies where the economic evaluation is being carried out alongside a randomised controlled trial (RCT), the resources that are required can be monitored prospectively, but when carried out in conjunction with a systematic review, it becomes more difficult, since costs are specific to a particular setting and country, while the studies are likely to have been undertaken in different settings and across many countries.

The most appropriate method for measuring productivity costs is subject to debate.[2,6] The *human capital approach* considers the value of potentially lost production resulting from a disease in terms of absenteeism, reduced productivity and disability or premature death at a specific age until the age of retirement. The human capital approach uses the gross wage rate as the measure to determine productivity losses caused by changes in paid working time resulting from health care programmes. The alternative, *friction cost method*, assumes that production losses are confined to the period needed to replace the 'sick' worker.[7]

These two approaches produce similar estimates when the health problem results in a short-term effect on productivity, but when long-term disability and mortality are the focus of attention, there can be significant differences between the two approaches. In reality the difference between the two approaches comes down to the valuation placed on non-work time and the costs of replacing workers, and when leisure time is highly valued relative to work time and there are significant replacement costs, the two approaches produce very similar estimates. A third approach to the measurement of productivity costs has been recommended in the USA by the Panel on

Cost-Effectiveness in Health and Medicine.[3] This approach assumes that part of the productivity impact of health problems is reflected in the health effects, and measured by some alternative approach to money, and also that to estimate the impact by using the wage rate would be to double-count the costs associated with productivity losses and gains.

In the UK, while the annual cost of absenteeism has been estimated at over 1% of GDP,[8] it is also known that health risk factors and disease adversely affect worker productivity.[9] For example, 3–11 hours per week in terms of productivity is lost to employers and 'because of presenteeism, previous reports of absenteeism may represent only a fraction of the cost of depression in the workplace'.[10] In a Canadian study it was demonstrated that most productivity loss days were a result of 'restricted days' rather than absenteeism per se.[11] In a US study, researchers found that lost productivity due to presenteeism was on average 7.5 times greater than productivity due to absenteeism, and for some conditions including migraine and neck/back/spine pain, the ratio was approaching 30:1.[12]

In the case of non-work activities the time spent in undertaking domestic responsibilities and participating in social and leisure activities is multiplied by an adjusted wage rate, either the take-home rate[2] or a multiple of the net wage rate.[13,14] It is important that these be included from a societal perspective, because these activities do have value and are sacrificed when having to attend health care facilities, or illness and disease preventing people from participating in them.

Valuation of costs

The final stage refers to the valuation of these resource effects. If prices exist for these effects and can be assumed to reflect costs, these can be multiplied by the relevant units of service to produce total costs, such as x bed days multiplied by £y per day.

In terms of productivity costs, differences in the approach to how they are measured can lead to highly significant differences in the valuation of costs. For example, the indirect non-medical costs of neck pain in the Netherlands in 1996 were estimated at $526.5 million, using the human capital approach and at $96.3 million using the friction cost method.[15] Similarly, the indirect cost of back pain in the UK was estimated at £10.7 billion, using the human capital approach and at £5 billion, using the friction cost method.[16]

Approaches to the measurement and valuation of costs

There are basically two approaches that can be employed in measuring resource inputs and attempting to value them – microcosting, or the bottom-up approach; and gross costing, or the top-down approach.[2,17] Microcosting refers to the detailed analysis of the changes in resource use due to the service or programme, similar in nature to time-and-motion studies. Such detailed, bottom-up, collection of data on resource use may be necessary when changes are being made to existing services (adding an extra stage or test). With microcosting, valuation use is also likely to require customised work, as prices are unlikely to be available. Although many analysts favour the bottom-up approach, it tends to be costly and runs the risk of being context-specific.

Gross costing allocates a total budget to the service, or alternatively considers the level of expenditure incurred by the service, and then divides by the number of patients to arrive at the cost per patient. The simplicity of the top-down approach may be offset by a lack of sensitivity, which in turn depends on the type of routine data available.

The approach employed to estimate the cost profile of health care services depends on the particular situation. For example, in a study to assess the costs associated with orthodontic provision in the UK, there are a number of issues that highlight the difficulties involved in accurately estimating the costs of health care provision, as compared to calculating the cost of producing widgets.[18] Ideally, costing orthodontic clinics would involve the estimation of salaries, services and overheads, with treatment costs based on the treatment times and overall duration of treatment. This was possible in relation to the salaried services, orthodontic provision in the hospital and community settings, but in the General Dental Services payment to practitioners is based on a 'fee for item' system. These fees are supposed to reflect the costs incurred by the practice. They also include a profit element, which at one level can be regarded as the necessary reward (and hence cost) to keep orthodontists in the service, but also as economic rent, which is the amount of money over and above what is actually necessary to keep orthodontists in practice. The use of fees and tariffs is not likely to represent the opportunity cost of that particular service and should only be used if there is a clear indication that a tariff or fee for service provided represents only a small proportion of the total cost of the service.[2]

Table 3.1 highlights the unit costs of health care professionals, derived from an annual publication produced by the Personal Social Services Research Unit at the University of Kent in Canterbury,[19] while Table 3.2 highlights the costs of treatments and procedures carried out in hospitals across England.[20]

It is worth noting the range of costs recorded in Table 3.2, as indicated by the interquartile range – a feature that highlights the difficulties in using published cost data for undertaking economic evaluations of health care interventions. The costs are based on Health Care Resource Groups (HRGs), which are a means of classifying the interventions, treatments and procedures carried out within hospitals. The intention is to establish tariffs for HRGs, which will mean that hospitals that can carry out the procedures at a rate below the tariff will gain financially while the opposite will occur in those hospitals that fail to provide at such a rate.

Table 3.1 Unit costs of health care professionals.

Professional	£/h of patient contact	£/surgery/clinic/patient related minute
General practitioner		
(including direct care staff costs)		
with qualification costs	127	2.09
without qualification costs	108	1.80
(excluding direct care staff costs)		
with qualification costs	116	1.91
without qualification costs	98	1.62
Prescription costs per consultation equivalent to £30.97		
Hospital physiotherapist		
with qualification costs	39	0.62
without qualification costs	35	0.55
Hospital pharmacist		
with qualification costs	54	0.65
without qualification costs	47	0.57
Medical consultant		
with qualification costs	109	1.82
without qualification costs	88	1.47
Psychiatric consultant		
with qualification costs	260	1.88
without qualification costs	210	1.52
Radiographer		
with qualification costs	47	0.80
without qualification costs	41	0.70
Staff nurse (24-h ward)		
with qualification costs	40	0.33
without qualification costs	35	0.28

Continued

Table 3.1—*Continued*

Professional	£/h of patient contact	£/surgery/clinic/patient related minute
Staff nurse (day ward)		
with qualification costs	32	0.3
without qualification costs	28	0.25
Specialist registrar		
with qualification costs	40	0.47
without qualification costs	27	0.32

Classification of costs

Fixed and variable costs

- *Fixed costs* arise no matter how many units of output or outcomes are produced.
- *Variable costs*, on the other hand, vary directly with output and cease to exist without service provision commencing or when service provision ceases.

However, when it has been shown that new techniques or practices can result in so-called savings in staff time, managers and finance staff are quick to point out that it is not possible to translate these into financial savings, because the salary costs are relatively fixed and can only be reduced by getting rid of staff. This has been evidenced in the employment of agency nurses to cover staff shortages on hospital wards. The agency nurses are actually paid more per hour than the full-time employed nurses, but the total cost of employment of the latter group is greater due to the fact that they are what may be termed *semi-fixed*, and therefore incur salary and on-costs compared to the variable nature of agency nurses, who are only employed for short periods of time, as and when required.

Total, average and marginal costs

- *Total costs* of an activity or a service are the sum of all expenditures (or the sum of all opportunity costs) during some specified period.
- *Average cost* is the total cost divided by the number of units provided or produced. When average costs are falling, there exist *economies of scale*; when average costs are rising, there exist *diseconomies of scale*. The initial economies are due to two factors: the sharply falling average fixed cost (e.g. the cost of running a hospital building is shared between increasing numbers of patients) and the falling average variable cost (e.g. the number of patients

Table 3.2 NHS reference costs.

HRG code	HRG label	No. of FCEs	Average unit cost (£)	Lower quartile (£)	Upper quartile (£)	No. of bed-days	Average length of stay
	ELECTIVE INPATIENTS						
E01	Heart and lung transplant	16	30 128	4 836	22 132	268	16.75
E02	Heart transplant	119	14 114	5 875	24 807	1 145	9.62
E03	Cardiac valve procedures	6 139	8 419	7 158	9 668	53 290	8.68
E04	Coronary bypass	15 184	6 320	2 453	6 836	103 598	6.82
E05	Other cardiothoracic procedures with cardiopulmonary support	3 002	5 349	964	4 606	15 971	5.32
E06	Other cardiothoracic procedures without cardiopulmonary support	1 239	4 083	1 871	5 030	4 943	3.99
E07	Pacemaker implant for AMI, heart failure or shock	108	4 400	1 533	4 587	466	4.31
E08	Pacemaker implant except for AMI, heart failure or shock	7 141	3 767	1 533	3 561	19 064	2.67
E09	Cardiac pacemaker replacement/revision	3 594	2 899	1 014	2 996	7 647	2.13
E10	Other circulatory procedures	1 426	1 917	905	2 674	5 132	3.60
E11	Acute myocardial infarction with cc	281	1 939	1 048	2 288	2 223	7.91
E12	Acute Myocardial Infarction without cc	498	1 523	872	1 719	2 692	5.41
E13	Cardiac catheterisation with complications	280	1 617	506	2 473	982	3.51
E14	Cardiac catheterisation without complications	15 355	1 254	755	1 592	36 218	2.36

Table 3.2—*Continued*

HRG code	HRG label	No. of FCEs	Average unit cost (£)	Lower quartile (£)	Upper quartile (£)	No. of bed-days	Average length of stay
E15	Percutaneous transluminal coronary angioplasty (PTCA)	15 547	2 827	1 381	3 254	25 960	1.67
E16	Other percutaneous cardiac procedures	5 137	2 240	1 133	2 473	9 604	1.87
E17	Endocarditis	60	3 495	1 255	5 123	889	14.82
E18	Heart failure or shock > 69 or with cc	1 158	2 131	1 328	2 796	15 047	12.99
E19	Heart failure or shock < 70 without cc	512	1 595	862	2 620	12 116	23.66
E20	Deep vein thrombosis > 69 or with cc	357	1 188	667	2 210	1 650	4.62
E21	Deep vein thrombosis < 70 without cc	399	686	542	1 834	884	2.22
E22	Coronary atherosclerosis > 69 or with cc	572	2 121	654	2 399	3 036	5.31
E23	Coronary atherosclerosis < 70 without cc	695	1 562	666	1 468	1 979	2.85
E24	Hypertension > 69 or with cc	232	1 451	690	2 189	1 256	5.41
E25	Hypertension < 70 without cc	372	938	491	1 279	1 111	2.99
E26	Congenital or valvular disorders > 69 or with cc	783	2 705	1 183	2 812	4 306	5.50
E27	Congenital or valvular disorders < 70 without cc	1 240	2 294	745	2 151	3 977	3.21
E28	Cardiac arrest	69	1 594	519	2 101	351	5.09
E29	Arrhythmia or conduction disorders > 69 or with cc	2 037	956	603	1 333	6 775	3.33
E30	Arrhythmia or conduction disorders < 70 without cc	1 752	728	351	986	3 328	1.90

Continued

Table 3.2—*Continued*

HRG code	HRG label	No. of FCEs	Average unit cost (£)	Lower quartile (£)	Upper quartile (£)	No. of bed-days	Average length of stay
E31	Syncope or collapse > 69 or with cc	354	1 370	605	1 778	1 943	5.49
E32	Syncope or collapse < 70 without cc	367	1 107	476	1 203	800	2.18
E33	Angina > 69 or with cc	875	1 582	779	1 907	4 124	4.71
E34	Angina < 70 without cc	814	1 362	587	1 379	2 554	3.14
E35	Chest pain > 69 or with cc	324	1 183	681	1 605	1 130	3.49
E36	Chest pain < 70 without cc	509	1 116	431	1 084	1 100	2.16
E37	Other cardiac diagnoses	1 590	1 477	650	1 719	6 207	3.90
E99	Complex elderly with a cardiac primary diagnosis	653	2 651	1 524	3 688	7 621	11.67
NON-ELECTIVE INPATIENTS							
E01	Heart and lung transplant	10	27 132	17 559	32 404	168	16.80
E02	Heart transplant	79	31 156	4 771	24 383	890	11.27
E03	Cardiac valve procedures	1 670	9 518	7 671	10 395	17 296	10.36
E04	Coronary bypass	4 746	6 867	3 144	7 302	37 021	7.80
E05	Other cardiothoracic procedures with cardiopulmonary support	2 109	4 583	1 234	4 638	18 073	8.57
E06	Other cardiothoracic procedures without cardiopulmonary support	878	3 681	1 507	4 476	5 185	5.91

Table 3.2—*Continued*

HRG code	HRG label	No. of FCEs	Average unit cost (£)	Lower quartile (£)	Upper quartile (£)	No. of bed-days	Average length of stay
E07	Pacemaker implant for AMI, heart failure or shock	923	3 271	1 173	3 644	8 157	8.84
E08	Pacemaker implant except for AMI, heart failure or shock	9 638	3 615	1 204	3 274	64 524	6.69
E09	Cardiac pacemaker replacement/revision	1 011	2 907	845	2 707	3 924	3.88
E10	Other circulatory procedures	3 853	2 210	1 230	3 042	29 862	7.75
E11	Acute myocardial infarction with cc	18 945	1 450	1 226	1 753	173 857	9.18
E12	Acute myocardial infarction without cc	74 478	955	790	1 197	663 454	8.91
E13	Cardiac catheterisation with complications	931	2 517	1 522	3 090	8 130	8.73
E14	Cardiac catheterisation without complications	21 362	1 990	1 168	2 155	759 017	35.53
E15	Percutaneous transluminal coronary angioplasty (PTCA)	15 733	3 141	853	3 092	49 032	3.12
E16	Other percutaneous cardiac procedures	2 131	1 963	887	2 109	10 305	4.84
E17	Endocarditis	1 271	2 800	1 643	3 611	18 310	14.41
E18	Heart failure or shock > 69 or with cc	56 907	1 516	1 281	1 769	706 849	12.42
E19	Heart failure or shock < 70 without cc	12 933	1 130	918	1 379	75 460	5.83
E20	Deep vein thrombosis > 69 or with cc	12 303	1 096	873	1 476	72 773	5.92
E21	Deep vein thrombosis < 70 without cc	11 870	736	548	1 091	39 376	3.32
E22	Coronary atherosclerosis > 69 or with cc	6 073	1 331	1 015	1 535	39 614	6.52

Continued

Table 3.2—*Continued*

HRG code	HRG label	No. of FCEs	Average unit cost (£)	Lower quartile (£)	Upper quartile (£)	No. of bed-days	Average length of stay
E23	Coronary atherosclerosis < 70 without cc	4 518	928	570	1 118	18 376	4.07
E24	Hypertension > 69 or with cc	3 088	1 068	796	1 266	17 197	5.57
E25	Hypertension < 70 without cc	3 559	712	511	995	10 276	2.89
E26	Congenital or valvular disorders > 69 or with cc	4 952	1 967	1 165	2 123	43 963	8.88
E27	Congenital or valvular disorders < 70 without cc	3 255	1 457	806	1 516	14 321	4.40
E28	Cardiac arrest	2 367	929	662	1 155	9 924	4.19
E29	Arrhythmia or conduction disorders > 69 or with cc	55 532	982	813	1 188	640 583	11.54
E30	Arrhythmia or conduction disorders < 70 without cc	33 656	536	426	707	120 217	3.57
E31	Syncope or collapse > 69 or with cc	46 895	885	738	1 151	335 772	7.16
E32	Syncope or collapse < 70 without cc	20 921	479	363	660	41 075	1.96
E33	Angina > 69 or with cc	74 409	797	652	1 018	499 829	6.72
E34	Angina < 70 without cc	60 794	605	453	798	200 400	3.30
E35	Chest pain > 69 or with cc	51 708	566	456	741	305 079	5.90
E36	Chest pain < 70 without cc	106 433	390	310	542	453 354	4.26
E37	Other cardiac diagnoses	14 779	1 068	814	1 252	69 590	4.71
E99	Complex elderly with a cardiac primary diagnosis	40 354	1 866	1 570	2 287	456 107	11.30

per nurse). One of the reasons diseconomies arise is because beyond a certain occupancy level it becomes increasingly difficult, if not impossible, for staff to deal with a larger number of beds in a ward setting.

- *Marginal cost* refers to the change in cost associated with a change in the level of activity. For example, the cost associated with increasing a community nurse's caseload by one additional patient may be relatively insignificant if the new patient is the spouse of a current patient and with relatively low care needs. On the other hand, the cost may be enormous if the patient requires intensive treatment and support and is living alone in extremely poor housing conditions in a remote location.

Differences between average and marginal costs

In measuring costs and benefits it is important to distinguish between marginal and average costs. Differences between them can be considerable and marginal costs can change dramatically as the scale of service provision changes. This is probably best illustrated by the oft-quoted example of the sixth stool guaiac test.[21] The American Cancer Society endorsed a protocol of six sequential stool tests (guaiacs) for cancer of the large bowel. Evidence suggested that about 6 cancers out of 10 000 would not be identified (false negatives) if only one test were done. The average cost of each cancer diagnosed was $1175. If six tests were done the number of false negatives would fall to 0.00003 and the average cost of each cancer diagnosed would increase to $2451. Six guaiac tests were therefore recommended to doctors as being best practice. Neuhauser and Lewicki demonstrated how average and marginal costs would change with each additional test; the results are summarised in Table 3.3. It is important to note that when comparing two alternative programmes for achieving an objective, it is the additional costs incurred and the additional benefits accrued from the new programme that are of interest. In other words, we are looking at the marginal costs and benefits of the new programme compared to the comparator programme.

Another factor is that average cost may not be an accurate reflection of reality. For example, the average cost of a hospital episode includes the relatively high levels of resource utilisation during the first few days and the lower hotel costs during the latter stages. Therefore the issue of whether to use marginal or average depends very much on the nature of the comparison and setting. For example, in a comparison of two anaesthetic programmes that require different types of infrastructure, average costs are recommended because the fixed cost element would be ignored by the use of marginal cost. However, when the choice is between two or more analgesics, the use of marginal cost rather than average would be more appropriate.[2]

Capital costs

These costs are incurred when major assets are acquired – the buildings, the equipment, etc. Capital costs are not merely the sum actually paid for their

Table 3.3 Costs of diagnosing bowel cancer and marginal cost of each additional cancer identified.

	Diagnosing bowel cancer			For each additional cancer identified		
Number of tests	Total cases detected	Total cost ($) million	Average cost ($) million	Extra cases detected	Extra costs ($) million	Marginal costs ($)
1	235 525	277	1175	235 525	277	1 175
2	255 152	385	1507	19 627	108	5 492
3	256 787	465	1811	1 625	80	49 000
4	256 924	529	2059	137	64	470 000
5	256 935	583	2268	11	54	4 700 000
6	256 936	630	2451	1	47	47 000 000

acquisition and the interest payments on any loans used to fund such purchases. Account also has to be taken of the opportunity cost of using such assets in one particular way, thereby depriving them of being used elsewhere. For example, long after the land, buildings and equipment have been paid for, there is a capital cost of continuing to use a hospital to provide health care, that is, as long as it could be used in an alternative way. For example, if the hospital could be sold, the opportunity cost would be its market value. There are many examples of ex-hospital sites now occupied by houses, with the street names the only visible indicator that a hospital was located there. However, it is usual to estimate the *equivalent annual cost* by annuitizing the initial capital outlay over the useful life of the asset. Therefore, if a piece of equipment costs £10 000 and has an expected life of 5 years, the equivalent annual cost is the sum that over the 5-year period will repay the £10 000 cost plus interest payments.

Joint costs
A further difficulty arises in the area of costs that are not unique to the project in question. For example, a hospital inpatient receives treatment, which involves inputs of medical staff, other staff, drugs, dressings, diagnostic tests, etc. but the hospital also incurs other costs in the form of maintenance of grounds and equipment, general management, cleaning and so on, which are reflected in the overall costs of the hospital. However, if the system of marginal costs is adhered to, only the additional resources required to treat the patient, or alternatively, the resources that will be released for the use of others, need be considered.

The problem with budgets

It has been suggested that because drug costs are easy to measure they are an 'obvious target for restrictions' and that 'we must resist the temptation to focus on easily measured drug costs while ignoring other major costs and sources of waste'.[22] However, the problem with many health care systems is that they are highly fragmented, and budgets, and the management of such, tend to exert a high degree of influence over decision-making. The consequences of decisions made in one area with regard to reducing drug costs, for example, have knock-on consequences in many other areas and impact perversely on numerous other budgets. In fact it has been shown in Canada that if all provinces increased drug spending to the levels observed in the two provinces with the highest spending level, an average of 584 fewer infant deaths and over 6 months of increased life expectancy at birth would result.[23]

It is important to remember that the cost of treatment is not only the cost of drugs or medical and nursing time but includes recovery times, incidence of side-effects, rate of delayed discharge, use of other care resources and the cost of system deficiencies and problems. It has been argued that the cost of system deficiencies and problems are much more expensive than drug costs[24] and 'it is important to remember that the cost to a facility of a 30-minute delay in the arrival of a surgeon is greater than the cost of a 2-hour infusion of propofol'.[25]

Obviously there are pressures within the health care system to ensure that expenditure levels do not exceed budgetary allocations. Hence, there are 'imperatives' to try and ensure that patients in high-cost areas, such as intensive care units, are transferred as quickly as possible to relatively lower-cost facilities, such as a high-dependency setting or a normal ward, obviously when judged clinically fit to do so. Similarly, much has been made in the press of delayed discharges from hospitals or what have become known as 'bed-blockers'. Patients classified by hospital consultants as ready for discharge, occupy beds that are required for other people on waiting lists. Delays in their discharge may occur because social services departments may not have funding available to set up an alternative package of care, or because of disagreements over who is responsible for continuing care. These patients become pawns in the interagency, interprofessional 'skirmishes' that then occur. Hospital staff and managers believe that the discharge of these patients is delayed, whereas social services departments argue that the discharge can only occur when all the necessary arrangements for continuing care have been made. However, what is apparent is that a patient occupying a bed 'unnecessarily' represents a 'waste of resources' from the perspective of the health service, while from the perspective of the social services department, no expenditure is being incurred. The Audit Commission[26] described the situation whereby agencies are 'locked in a vicious circle in which it is becoming increasingly difficult to free up the resources for alternative services that might ease the pressure'. It is not difficult to recognise both the irony and irrationality of the situation. People deemed suitable for discharge can be provided with the relevant treatment and care in facilities that are generally less expensive than acute hospital wards. However, because of these inter-agency and interprofessional 'disputes' limited resources are far from being used efficiently.

There is at least one aspect to bear in mind in analysing such situations. The unit of account, or unit of expenditure, is not the patient as such but the particular hospital episode, referred to as 'finished consultant episode', or the package of care. Thus, the patient who leaves an intensive care setting and moves to a normal ward also moves to the care of another consultant and to another budget. The patient who leaves hospital and is transferred to care in the community also moves to another budget. It does not matter whether such a person has to be readmitted to hospital or retransferred to intensive care, having been discharged from hospital or transferred from intensive care prematurely or inappropriately. For example, if we take the case of the patient in intensive care from a budgetary perspective:

> 3 days in intensive care, followed by 2 days in a ward, another 3 days in intensive care, then 5 days in a ward

is preferable to

> 4 days in intensive care followed by 7 days in a ward.

In the first scenario there are two intensive care episodes and two ward episodes, each of which has a shorter length of stay than the two episodes – one in intensive care and one in the ward – of the second scenario. If we assume that the cost per day of an intensive care bed is £1000 and the cost per bed-day in a ward is £200, the overall cost of the first scenario is £7400 (£3000 + £400 + £3000 + £1000) compared with £5400 (£4000 + £1400) for the second scenario.

Another example of the problems created by the budget-focused decision-making process was clearly highlighted in a study carried out in Hong Kong to assess the cost-effectiveness of intravenous ketorolac and morphine for treating pain after limb injury. The unit cost of ketorolac was nearly three times as expensive as morphine – HK$7.53 (£0.52) compared to HK$2.81 (£0.19). However, the mean overall cost per person amounted to HK$43.60 (£2.99) for those in the ketorolac group and HK$228.80 (£15.68) in the morphine group ($p < 0.0001$), with much of the difference between the two groups accounted for by the management of adverse events.[27]

Iatrogenic costs

A narrow budget-focused approach also fails to grasp the nature and extent of iatrogenic costs that result from health care interventions and services. As a result, they are not included as part of the decision-making process, and yet they can prove to be highly significant. For example, the costs and long-term health problems resulting from hospital-acquired infection (HAI) have been highlighted, with governments introducing policies to reduce the problem and the resources utilised in treating patients who suffer from the problem. The annual cost of HAI in England alone was estimated to be nearly £1 billion,[28] while an unpublished study with which the author was involved showed that surgical patients in Wales with infection stayed in hospital for, on average, 2 weeks more than those with no infection, at an excess cost of £3000 per patient. Recent initiatives to reduce the incidence of methicillin-resistant Staphylococcus aureus (MRSA) is at one level encouraging but also begs the question as to why it took so long for the problem to be tackled.[29]

Other examples of iatrogenic costs are to be found in the area of medicines management. A report by the Audit Commission[30] suggested that a large proportion of the £90 million worth of medicines that are taken each year into hospital by patients are thrown away. Another finding from the same study was that adverse events cost the NHS about £500 million a year for additional days spent by patients in hospital. The prevalence of adverse drug events detected by a retrospective record review in two acute hospitals was 6.5% of all hospital admissions and in 80% of cases it was the direct cause of admission. The cost of such admissions was estimated to be £466 million per year.[31] Another study reported that adverse drug events in UK hospitals cost the NHS £380 million a year – which in health currency units represents 15–20 400-bed hospitals.[32]

It has also been estimated that one in every eight patients admitted to hospitals in England and Wales each year experiences preventable adverse events, leading to an additional 3 million bed-days at a cost to the NHS of £1 billion a year. In other words, the NHS incurs an expenditure of £500 million on events and situations that could have been avoided.[33] Adverse events occurred in 17% of hospital admissions in Australia, half of which were considered preventable and which cost A$4.7 billion a year.[34] In the USA, 4% of hospital admissions led to adverse events, resulting in permanent disability in 7% and contributing to death in 14% of cases,[35,36] while in the UK one-third of adverse events led to at least moderate disability or death.[33]

Box 3.3 The Cost of NSAIDs

There are about 24 million prescriptions written for non-steroidal anti-inflammatory drugs (NSAIDs) per year in the UK, with the majority given to patients aged over 60. They are important and effective in the control of acute pain, chronic pain and in moderate to severe post-operative pain. The benefits of aspirin, for example, in preventing cardiovascular events are well known, while there is also evidence for its effectiveness in reducing the incidence and mortality from colon cancer.

Continued

Box 3.3 The Cost of NSAIDs—*Continued*

However, NSAIDs are important causes of upper gastrointestinal (GI) ulceration and dyspeptic symptoms, and in order to reduce risk acid-suppressing medication is often co-prescribed, with proton pump inhibitors (PPIs) increasingly the drug of choice. In 2000, there were 23 million prescriptions for ulcer-healing drugs at a net ingredient cost of £540 million in the UK. It has been estimated that for a primary care group of 100 000 patients the costs of co-prescribing might be in excess of £500 000 per year, depending on the extent of co-prescribing and the medication used, which translates to over £300 million per year across the NHS. In addition to these prescribing costs must be added the considerable human and economic burden associated with NSAID-induced GI disease. From the case notes of all emergency admissions for upper GI crises to two district general hospitals with a combined catchment population of 550 000, it was estimated that some 12 000 emergency upper GI admissions were attributable to NSAID use and that over 2200 deaths in hospitals and another 330 in the community could be attributed to NSAID use each year. Another study concluded that on average 1 in 1220 patients taking oral NSAIDs for 2 months or more dies due to GI complications.

Therefore, a major dilemma confronts those who have to determine patient treatment regimens. NSAIDs are highly effective analgesics, provide protection against cardiovascular events and have other potential benefits, but also lead to a three- to tenfold increase in ulcer complications, hospitalisation and death. In addition, it has been reported that NSAIDs were responsible for approximately 19% of hospital admissions with congestive heart failure (CHF), and led the authors to conclude that the burden of illness resulting from NSAID-related CHF may exceed that resulting from GI tract damage.

They also know that PPIs are highly effective gastro-protective agents and effective in the healing and maintenance of NSAID-induced ulcers. This dilemma exists against the background of limited resources and pressures to contain budgets, to prescribe generically and at the lowest possible cost. But the question that needs to be addressed is cost to whom?

Source: Phillips.[37]

One area that has received considerable attention is the iatrogenic costs associated with non-steroidal anti-inflammatory drug (NSAID) prescribing highlighted in Box 3.3.

The iatrogenic costs associated with NSAIDs in the UK have been estimated at between £32 and £70 for each patient prescribed an NSAID, and the total effect on the NHS was estimated to be between £166 million and £367 million per year.[38] In Sweden estimates of NSAID-induced gastric side-effects range from SKr320 million to SKr589 million;[39] in the Netherlands, they range between €39 million and €98 million;[40] and in Quebec (Canada), approximately CAN$1 would be added to patient costs for every day a patient was on NSAID therapy.[41]

Other factors that inflate costs of health care provision

In addition to the costs resulting from the adverse effects of treatment, there are other costs that result in limited resources being used wastefully. For example, many people fail to comply with their treatment requirements. This is very evident in relation to prescribed medicines. It is known, for example, that at the year ending, 31 March 2002, 609 tonnes of medicines were incinerated in the UK under the 'Disposal of old pharmaceuticals' scheme. This was a 59% rise over the preceding 4 years although, in the same period, the number of prescription items dispensed rose by only 20%. Estimates have placed the financial value of medicines that are not used in the UK between £30 million and £90 million per annum, but these are mostly based on extrapolations of medicines returned to community pharmacies and are likely be gross underestimates.[42] In addition, over one-third of patients with chronic conditions do not take their medicines as prescribed.[43] Whether lack of compliance results in increased costs is subject to debate, but one study estimated that the cost associated with non-compliance was DM10 billion per year.[44]

There are also the unnecessary consultations that result from inappropriate and ineffective treatments being utilised. For example, in the treatment of gastro-oesoephageal reflux disease, it was shown that the total cost of a stepped approach to treatment (a trial-and-error strategy, where the patient is told to try a treatment and 'come back and see me if it does not work' scenario) amounted to £224 000 compared to £185 000 for a relatively high-cost but effective treatment, which resulted in fewer consultations.[45]

A similar situation was shown to exist when the use of an expensive but effective procedure resulted in fewer inappropriate surgical procedures and adjuvant radiotherapy and chemotherapy regimens from being used in patients with rectal cancer than existing clinical practice.[46]

There are also the costs resulting from litigation and claims for damages following treatment and care, which have gone wrong. It is acknowledged that we live in an age where the threat of litigation has increased substantially – for example, the bill for negligence claims against the NHS in England was £84 million in 1998,[47] but by March 2000 the provision to meet likely settlements for outstanding claims was £2.6 billion, with a further £1.3 billion to meet likely settlements for claims expected to arise from incidents that had occurred but not been reported.[48] It is not surprising therefore that the Audit Commission offered the following view:

In recent years, these cost pressures have been driven by the introduction of new medicines. . . . These cost pressures are cause for concern for many Trust boards, but they need to be viewed as part of the overall package of patient care. For some conditions, medicines expenditure should be rising because it would be a cost-effective way of increasing the health gain for the population. For example, expenditure on proton pump inhibitors and H2 antagonists should be rising because their use improves the quality of patients' lives and saves money by preventing invasive surgery.[30]

It is the aggregation of these iatrogenic costs that indicate the extent to which resources are not being used as efficiently as they might in seeking to maximise the health benefits for society. However, what is noticeable is that the focus of attention in managing resources is primarily on the costs that are easily observed and the 'iceberg effect' is often ignored. Decisions are often made on the basis of the costs that are visible, above the water, while those that lie below the water, and are often of considerable magnitude, do not enter the decision-making process.

It has been pointed out in the case of pain management that policymakers need to be fully aware of all aspects associated with the costs of pain and its management:

- costs of interventions and therapies for treating pain and securing pain relief (e.g. drug costs and staff costs);
- costs that are incurred as a result of ineffective interventions being provided (e.g. costs of additional GP consultations);
- costs to health service and patients and their families due to lack of appropriate facilities within locality (e.g. costs of accessing alternative therapies);
- costs resulting from inappropriate self-medication and treatment by patients (e.g. costs of treating overdoses);
- costs of treating and preventing adverse events that arise as a result of prescribing decisions (e.g. costs of GI bleeds);
- costs of disability claims resulting from people's inability to work (incapacity benefits and the like are regarded as transfer payments and represent a cost to the government but a gain to the recipient, with a neutral overall impact on society. However, in an environment of constraints on levels of public expenditure, the opportunity cost associated with increasing benefits expenditure can be significant, while the long-term effect of inactivity and reliance on benefits can result in severe social problems);
- costs to economy of reductions in productivity and absenteeism (the different approaches to measuring productivity costs have been discussed earlier);
- costs of providing social care and support to people suffering with pain (e.g. costs of home care and respite care);
- costs of informal care provided by families (e.g. loss of earnings);

- costs of intangibles associated with deterioration in the QOL of patients and their families.

The argument was made that the burden of suffering that pain imposes on individuals, and the enormous costs that society has to bear as a result necessitate that policymakers and decision-makers alike should adopt a much wider, strategic perspective in their deliberations regarding service provision and resource allocation.[49]

Cost of illness studies

Cost of illness or burden of illness studies aim to assess the overall economic effects of illness and disease on individuals, the health service, the economy and society. They serve as points of reference for economic analyses[50] and are useful in highlighting the impact that illnesses and diseases have on health services and societies. They have been widely used by organisations such as the WHO and the World Bank, but as has been pointed out, policymakers should not be misled into thinking that 'cost of illness' studies provide suitable evidence in determining whether more resources should be devoted to a given disease. 'These issues can only be addressed by considering the costs and effectiveness of interventions for the disease in question.'[13]

There are a number of approaches and indicators used to assess the burden of illness. For example, the prevalence of a disease is used to estimate the costs for that disease during a period of time. The cost of coronary artery disease in the UK was estimated by using the number of prevalent cases and aggregated data relating to mortality, morbidity and health service utilisation. In addition, a societal perspective was employed by including both direct and productivity costs. The direct health care costs were estimated at £1.8 billion and the productivity costs of the disease were estimated at £6.7 billion, using the human capital approach, and at £701 million, using the friction cost approach.[51]

Another example is taken from the condition asthma and its management. In 2001 it was estimated that 5.1 million people of all ages and social backgrounds were being treated for asthma in the UK (including 1.4 million children under 16 years of age) at a total annual cost to the UK health care system of over £850 million.[52] However, it is not the costs directly related to treatment that contribute the largest proportion to overall cost, but rather the costs of inappropriate treatments and non-compliance that result in suboptimal control and an excessive number of exacerbations and attacks resulting in hospitalisations. On average, in the UK the total health service costs are 3.53 times higher in patients who experience asthma attacks compared with those who do not,[53] while an Australian study demonstrated that the annual cost of a poorly controlled patient was A$4909 (£2168) compared with A$2094 (£925, 1991 prices) for a well-controlled patient.[54] A US study showed that the annual cost of a poorly controlled asthma patient was $7030 (£4594) compared with $47 (£31, 1994 prices) for a well-controlled patient,[55] and it is probable that half of all costs associated with asthma may be expected to arise from the one-fifth of patients who experience an attack.[53]

An alternative approach to estimating the burden of disease is to catalogue the lifetime costs based on the incidence of a condition. For example, the discounted costs to health and social services of providing treatment and care within the UK for a stroke survivor at 30 days have been estimated at £15 000 over a 5-year period and £24 000 over a lifetime (£17 000 and £34 000 when costs are not discounted).[56] In Canada, the lifetime cost per patient suffering with multiple sclerosis was estimated to be $1 148 570 (€1 320 197, 1995 prices).[57]

Another method employed has been to calculate the impact of disease on resources within the NHS. For example, it was estimated that primary care management of patients with chronic pain accounts for 4.6 million appointments per year in the UK, equivalent to 793 whole-time GPs, at a total cost of around £69 million.[58] Similarly, reference was made earlier to adverse drug events in UK hospitals, which in resource terms were equivalent to 15–20 400 bed hospitals.[32] It is this sort of interpretation that is picked up by the media, an example of which is provided in Box 3.4.

The WHO approach to estimating the burden of disease is to calculate the impact of illness on disability-adjusted life years (DALYs), which are the present value of future years of lifetime lost through premature mortality plus the present value of the adjustment to years of future lifetime to allow for the average severity (frequency and intensity) of any mental or physical disability caused by a disease or injury.[59] Work undertaken on behalf of the WHO has provided a clear demarcation between those diseases that have the greatest impact in developed countries and those that result in the greatest

---

Box 3.4 How the Media Portray Cost of Illness

In an editorial in *The Independent* (7 October 2004) entitled 'Sloth, gluttony and our rising rates of diabetes', it was reported that 'in Britain alone, 1.8 million people have been diagnosed and a further 1 million are thought to be living with the condition (i.e. diabetes) in ignorance that they have it. The numbers affected have more than doubled since 1980 and are set to almost double again by 2010, to 3 million. These are figures to make the eyes water. Already the NHS is spending £1 in every 20 on diabetes and its complications. By 2011, that is projected to rise to £1 in every 10. Can we afford it? And what other parts of health care will have to shrink as a result?'

number of DALYs lost in developing countries.[60] In developed countries the top ten causes of DALYs lost (percentage of total in parentheses) are:
(1) Ischaemic heart disease (9.9)
(2) Unipolar major depression (6.1)
(3) Cerebrovascular disease (5.9)
(4) Road traffic accidents (4.4)
(5) Alcohol use (4.0)
(6) Osteoarthritis (2.9)
(7) Trachea, bronchus and lung cancers (2.9)
(8) Dementia and other degenerative and hereditary central nervous system disorders (2.4)
(9) Self-inflicted injuries (2.3)
(10) Congenital abnormalities (2.2)

In developing countries the top ten diseases are:
(1) Lower respiratory infections (9.1)
(2) Diarrhoeal diseases (8.1)
(3) Conditions arising during the perinatal period (7.3)
(4) Unipolar major depression (3.4)
(5) Tuberculosis (3.1)
(6) Measles (3.0)
(7) Malaria (2.6)
(8) Ischaemic heart disease (2.5)
(9) Congenital abnormalities (2.4)
(10) Cerebrovascular disease (2.4)

The differences between regions of the world are also marked when the percentage of DALYs lost by age is compared. In sub-Saharan Africa over 50% of the burden is due to mortality and morbidity in the 0–4 age group, while for the leading developed countries in the world a similar percentage of DALYS lost is in the 45+ age group.[59,60] However, the use of DALYs as a measure of burden of illness is not without its problems, and further discussion on this point is provided in Chapter 4.

The impact of diseases on the QOL of patients and their families is a popular technique, with many examples in the literature. It is clear that an osteoporotic fracture has a major impact on a person's QOL over and above the effect of the trauma and pain. It has been reported that 12 months after a hip fracture[61,62]:

- 40% of patients are unable to walk independently;
- 60% are limited in at least one class I activity of daily living (e.g. feeding, dressing, toileting);
- 80% are limited in a class II activity of daily living (e.g. shopping, gardening, climbing stairs);
- 14% require nursing home care (after 12 months), although during the 12-month period, up to 27% of patients require nursing home care and 30% require some degree of home care support.

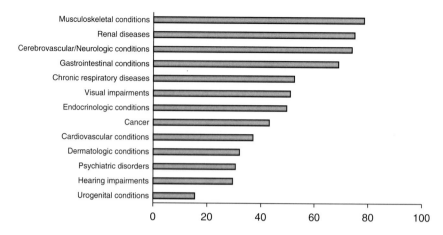

Figure 3.1 Impact of diseases on quality of life (QOL).

While there is an abundance of studies on individual disease areas, there is very little comparison of the relative impact of diseases on QOL. One such study is a systematic literature review of 20 studies that compared the QOL across chronic disease populations. To enable a comparison across conditions, they were aggregated into disease clusters and the relative position of each disease cluster was then established across studies in terms of its impact on QOL.[63] The results are shown in Figure 3.1; the disease cluster with the highest score has the greatest negative impact on QOL.

In the UK, a series of National Service Frameworks (NSFs) in a number of disease areas* have been formulated. If these NSFs are successful in reducing the extent and burden of disease, the argument is made that we would be able to 'save' a large percentage of the resources currently used in their treatment. However, the results from cost of illness studies do need to be treated with considerable caution. It has rightly been argued that they 'add little to the creation of an efficient health care system'.[64] In addition, they tend to focus on one condition and on issues specific to that condition. A recent Canadian study has shown that the number of diseases is a significant indicator of utilisation of health care services – an additional chronic disease is associated with 1.74 more physician visits per year in people under 60 years of age and 1.29 more physician visits in people aged 60 years and above.[65]

---

* National Service Frameworks are currently available in:
    Coronary heart disease
    Mental health
    Diabetes
    Children's services
    The care of the elderly
Further information relating to these is available at:
http://www.dh.gov.uk

Health economics is not only about the monetary benefits that result, and accountants and managers are always ready to point to the difficulties involved in translating so-called 'savings' into practice. However, the reduction in deaths and improvements in people's QOL resulting from the reduction in disease prevalence are highly significant, and while it may not be possible or indeed necessary to translate these into monetary values, they nevertheless represent highly important outcomes emerging from the successful implementation of the NSFs in the disease areas.

The important question from the perspective of health economics, however, is whether the resources channelled into one particular disease area might have produced 'better results' if used elsewhere. Chapter 2 explores the approaches to the identification, measurement and valuation of the outputs and outcomes resulting from health care programmes and interventions, in order to assess whether in fact 'better results' might be returned from the use of resources in other areas.

References

1 McPake B, Kumaranayake L, Normand C. Health Economics. *An international perspective*. London: Routledge, 2002.

2 Brouwer W, Rutten F, Koopmanschap M. Costing in economic evaluation, in Drummond MF, McGuire A (eds). *Economic evaluation in health care: merging theory with practice*. Oxford: Oxford University Press, 2001.

3 Sculpher M. The role and estimation of productivity costs in economic evaluation, in Drummond MF, McGuire A (eds). *Economic evaluation in health care: merging theory with practice*. Oxford: Oxford University Press, 2001.

4 Luce BR, Manning WG, Siegl JE *et al*. Estimating costs in cost-effectiveness analsyis, in Gold MR, Siegl JE, Russell LB *et al*. (eds). *Cost-effectiveness in health and medicine*. New York: Oxford University Press, 1996.

5 Phillips CJ. The cost of eczema: a UK perspective. *Dermatol Pract* 2002; 10: 22–24.

6 Drummond MF. Cost-of-illness studies: a major headache? *Pharmacoeconomics* 1992; 2: 1–4.

7 Koopmanschap MA, Rutten FFH, van Ineveld BM *et al*. The friction cost method for measuring indirect costs of disease. *J Health Econ* 1995; 14: 171–89.

8 Chatterji M, Tilley CJ. Sickness, absenteeism, presenteeism and sick pay. *Oxf Econ Papers* 2002; 54: 669–87.

9 Burton WN, Conti DJ, Chen CY *et al*. The role of health risk factors and disease on worker productivity. *J Occup Environ Med* 1999; 41: 863–77.

10 Druss BG, Rosenheck RA, Sledge WH. Health and disability costs of depression in a major U.S. Corporation. *Am J Psych* 2000; 157: 1274–78.

11 Ungar WJ, Coyte PC, The Pharmacy Medication Monitoring Program Advisory Board. Measuring productivity loss days in asthma patients. *Health Econ* 2000; 9: 37–46.

12 Main CJ, Phillips CJ, Watson PJ. Secondary prevention in health care and occupational settings in musculoskeletal conditions focusing on low back pain, in Schultz I, Gatchel RJ (eds). *Handbook of Complex Occupational Disability Claims*. New York: Springer, 2005.

13 Ratcliffe J, Ryan M, Tucker J. The costs of alternative types of routine antenatal care for low-risk women: shared care v care by general practitioners and community midwives. *J Health Serv Res Policy* 1996; 1: 135–40.

14 Posnet J, Jan S. Indirect cost in economic evaluation: the opportunity cost of unpaid input. *Health Econ* 1996; 5: 13–24.

15 Borghouts JAJ, Koes BW, Vondeling H *et al.* Cost-of-illness of neck pain in The Netherlands in 1996. *Pain* 1999; 80: 629–36.

16 Maniadakis N, Gray A. The economic burden of back pain in the UK. *Pain* 2000; 84: 95–103.

17 Raftery J. Economics notes: costing in economic evaluation. *BMJ* 2000; 320: 1597.

18 Richmond S, Durning P, Phillips CJ *et al.* The cost of the orthodontic service. *Orthodontics* 2004; 1: 255–62.

19 Curtis L, Netten A. *Unit Costs of Health and Social Care 2004.* Canterbury: Personal Social Services Research Unit, University of Kent. *http://www.pssru.ac.uk/pdf/uc2004/uc2004.pdf* (accessed 29 January 2004)

20 Department of Health. *NHS Reference Costs 2003. http://www.dh.gov.uk/assetRoot/04/07/01/10/04070110.xls* (accessed 29 January 2004)

21 Neuhauser A, Lewicki AM. What do we gain from the sixth stool guaic? *N Engl J Med* 1975; 293: 226–28.

22 Smith I. Cost considerations in the use of anaesthetic drugs. *Pharmacoeconomics* 2001; 19: 469–81.

23 Cremieux PY, Meilleur MC, Ouellette P *et al.* Public and private pharmaceutical spending as determinants of health outcomes in Canada. *Health Econ* 2004; 14: 107–16.

24 White PF, Watcha MF. Pharmacoeconomics in anaesthesia: what are the issues? *Eur J Anaesthesiol* 2001; 18(Suppl): 10–15.

25 Broadway PJ, Jones JG. A method of costing anaesthetic practice. *Anaesthesia* 1995; 50: 56–63.

26 Audit Commission. *Coming of Age.* London: Audit Commission, 1997.

27 Rainer TH, Jacobs P, Ng YC *et al.* Cost effectiveness analysis of intravenous ketorolac and morphine for treating pain after limb injury: double blind randomised controlled trial. *BMJ* 2000; 321: 1–9.

28 Plowman R, Graves N, Griffin M *et al. Socio-economic burden of hospital acquired infection.* London: Public Health Laboratory Service, 2000.

29 National Audit Office. *Improving patient care by reducing the risk of hospital acquired infection: a progress report.* London: Report by the Comptroller and Auditor General HC876, July 2004.

30 Audit Commission. *A spoonful of sugar: medicines management in NHS hospitals.* London: Audit Commission, 2001.

31 Pirmohamed M, James S, Meakin S *et al.* Adverse drug reactions as cause of admission to hospital: prospsective analysis of 18820 patients. *BMJ* 2004; 329: 15–19.

32 Wiffen P, Gill M, Edwards J *et al.* Adverse drug reactions in hospital patients: a systematic review of the prospective and retrospective studies. *Bandolier Extra* 2002; June.

33 Vincent C, Neale G, Woloshynowych M. Adverse events in British hospitals: preliminary retrospective record review. *BMJ* 2001; 322: 517–19.

34 Wilson RM, Runciman WB, Gibberd RW *et al.* The quality in Australian health care study. *Med J Aust* 1995; 163: 458–71.

35 Brennan TA, Leape LL, Laird NM *et al*. Incidence of adverse events and negligence in hospitalised patients. *N Engl J Med* 1991; 324: 370–76.

36 Leape LL, Brennan TA, Laird NM *et al*. Incidence of adverse events and negligence in hospitalised patients: results of the Harvard medical practice study II. *N Engl J Med* 1991; 324: 377–84.

37 Phillips CJ. And all because the doctor prescribed a NSAID: expenditure on PPIs and joined-up thinking in prescribing. *Br J Health Care Manag* 2002; 8: 272–75.

38 Moore RA, Phillips CJ. Cost of NSAID adverse effects to the UK National Health Service. *J Med Econ* 1999; 2: 45–55.

39 Jonsson B, Haglund U. Economic burden of NSAID-induced gastropathy in Sweden. *Scand J Gastroenterol* 2001; 36: 775–79.

40 Herings RM, Klungel OH. An epidemiological approach to assess the economic burden of NSAID-induced gastrointestinal events in The Netherlands. *Pharmacoeconomics* 2001; 19: 655–65.

41 Rahme E, Joseph L, Kong SX *et al*. Cost of prescribed NSAID-related gastrointestinal adverse events in elderly patients. *Br J Clin Pharmacol* 2001; 52: 185–92.

42 Mackridge A, Marriott J. When medicines are wasted so much is lost: to society as well as patients. *Pharmaceut J* 2004; 272: 12.

43 Marinker M, Blenkinsopp A, Bond C *et al*. (eds). *From compliance to concordance: achieving shared goals in medicine taking.* London: Royal Pharmaceutical Society of Great Britian, 1997.

44 Volmer T, Kielhorn A. Kosten der Non-Compliance. *Gesundh Oekon Qual Manag* 1999; 4: 55–61.

45 Phillips CJ, Moore RA. Trial and error – an expensive luxury: economic analysis of effectiveness of proton pump inhibitors and histamine antagonists in treating reflux disease. *Br J Med Econ* 1997; 11: 55–63.

46 Brown G, Davies S, Williams GT *et al*. Effectiveness of preoperative staging in rectal cancer: digital rectal examination, endoluminal ultrasound, or magnetic resonance imaging? *Br J Cancer* 2004; 5: 23–29.

47 Fenn P, Diacon S, Gray A *et al*. Current cost of medical negligence in NHS hospitals: analysis of claims database. *BMJ* 2000; 320: 1567–71.

48 National Audit Office. *Handling clinical negligence claims in England. Report by the Comptroller and Auditor General, HC403.* Session 2000–2001: 3 May 2001. London: HMSO, 2001.

49 Phillips CJ. The real cost of pain management. *Anaesthesia* 2001; 56: 1031–33.

50 Kobelt G. *Health economics: an introduction to economic evaluation.* London: Office of Health Economics, 2002.

51 Shearer A, Scuffham P, Mollon P. The cost of coronary artery disease in the UK. *Br J Cardiol* 2004; 11: 218–23.

52 National Asthma Campaign. Out in the open: a true picture of asthma in the United Kingdom today. National Asthma Campaign Asthma Audit 2001. *Asthma J* 2001; 6(Suppl).

53 Hoskins G, McCowan C, Neville RG *et al*. Risk factors and costs associated with an asthma attack. *Thorax* 2000; 55: 19–24.

54 National Asthma Campaign. *Report on the cost of asthma in Australia.* www.nationalasthma.org.au/publications/costs/costindx.html (last accessed 9 June 2003)

55 Johnson KA, Ernst RL, Ogostalick AE. Analysis of direct, indirect, and total costs of asthma from patient survey data. *Value Health* 2000; 2: 142–62.

56 Chambers M, Hutton J, Gladman J. Cost-effectiveness analysis of antiplatelet therapy in the prevention of recurrent stroke in the UK. *Pharmacoeconomics* 1999; 16: 577–93.

57 The Canadian Burden of Illness Study Group. Burden of illness of multiple sclerosis: Part I – cost of illness. *Can J Neurol Sci* 1998; 25: 23–30.

58 Belsey J. Primary care workload in the management of chronic pain: a retrospective cohort study using a GP database to identify resource implications for UK primary care. *J Med Econ* 2002; 5: 39–52.

59 Fox-Rushby J. *Disability-adjusted life years (DALYs) for decision-making? An overview of the literature.* London: Office of Health Economics, 2002.

60 Murray JL, Lopez AD (eds). *The global burden of disease: a comprehensive assessment of mortality and disability from diseases, injuries and risk factors in 1990 and projected to 2020.* Cambridge, MA: Harvard University Press, 1996.

61 Eastell R, Reid DM, Compston J *et al.* Secondary prevention of osteoporosis: when should a non-vertebral facture be a trigger for action? *Q J Med* 2001; 94: 575–97.

62 Cooper C. The crippling consequences of fractures and their impact on quality of life. *Am J Med* 1997; 103(Suppl): 12S–19S.

63 Sprangers MAG, de Regt EB, Andries F *et al.* Which chronic conditions are associated with a better or poorer quality of life? *J Clin Epidemiol* 2000; 53: 895–97.

64 Byford S, Torgerson DJ, Raftery J. Cost of illness studies. *BMJ* 2000; 320: 1335.

65 Rapoport J, Jacobs P, Bell NR *et al.* Refining the measurement of the economic burden of chronic diseases in Canada. *Chronic Dis Can* 2004; 25: 13–22. *http://www.phac-aspc.gc.ca/publicat/cdic-mcc/25–1/c_e.html* (accessed 24 January 2004)

CHAPTER 4
The benefits of health care: outputs and outcomes

The issues involved in attempting to determine the costs of providing health care services and in estimating the costs to society resulting from various diseases and illnesses were considered in Chapter 3. It concluded with a brief reference to the NSFs, each of which has established a series of service standards and targets to which professionals and decision-makers aspire in relation to securing improvements in people's health. The aim of this chapter is to consider what is meant by health care benefits, how they can be identified and described, and how they can be measured and used to assess the effectiveness and efficiency of health care interventions and programmes.

There are many difficulties involved in seeking to describe what constitutes health care benefits. For example, the incongruity of benefits resulting from health care provision was vividly expressed by a former professor of obstetrics and gynaecology, who reported that his role had involved 'saving babies one moment, killing them the next'. He expressed the view that

> medical technology has advanced to the point where it is possible for an emergency caesarean to save the life of a baby at 24 weeks of gestation with a good chance of it surviving perfectly normally. Yet while a foetus is being saved in one operating theatre, a termination for 'social reasons' may well be taking place in the next theatre on a foetus at exactly the same stage of development. (*Sunday Times* 4 July 2004)

What constitutes health benefits?

In any given health care situation there is a multiplicity of possible outcomes, the significance of which is dependent on the perspective being considered – that of the patient, the professional, the manager, the funding agency or any other stakeholder. The professional could provide the most perfect remedy for a clinical problem, but it will not, in itself, translate into an effective outcome if it is not 'owned' by patients, who are prepared to fully comply with the requirements of their treatment regimen. It is well recognised that the effectiveness of interventions is highly dependent upon compliance and adherence rates, and the issue of patient concordance is one which is increasingly being considered in attempts to elevate levels of treatment effectiveness in clinical practice to those of treatment efficacy achieved in clinical trials. Non-compliance can have major implications for both resource management and the management of the patient's condition,[1] emphasising the need for patients to be involved in treatment decisions. It has been advocated, for instance, that increasing the role of asthma nurses and the development of simpler treatment regimens with reduced dosing frequency and fewer inhalers would result in increased patient adherence and result in improved symptom control.[2]

Another consideration to bear in mind in a discussion of the benefits, results and consequences of health care service provision relates to the nature, extent and quality of the evidence available to support the decisions that are made. It has been argued that 'in the twenty-first century, the health care decision-maker, that is, anyone who makes decisions about groups of patients or populations, will have to practise evidence-based decision-making'.[3] Evidence-based decision-making, accordingly, is the ability to do the right things right. The evolution of evidence-based health care (EBHC) in the UK context can be traced from the 1970s when economic pressures initiated an era when cost issues became significant factors for health care decision-makers ('doing things cheaper'), through the quality initiatives of the 1980s ('doing things better') to the period when these were combined into the era of 'doing things right'.[3] Decision-makers have been provided with a framework (based around focusing on interventions that do good, stopping those that do harm and developing research to assess the effectiveness of those known to have an unknown effect) which influences not only how they practise but also what they practise.[3]

It is likely in the short-term future, at least, that there will be greater attempts to bridge the divide between research carried out in academic communities and the use of these findings by politicians and policymakers, with the questions not being restricted to
• What works?
but also including
• When does it work?
• Why does it work?
• Where does it work?
• How does it work?
• Under what circumstances does it work?
and summed up under a developed slogan of:
Doing the right things right for the right people at the right time under the right conditions.

Outputs and outcomes in health care services

However, in attempting to determine what the right things, the right time and the right conditions are, a distinction has to be made between outputs and outcomes. An output has been defined as 'a measurable product attributable to an input or combination of inputs', whereas an outcome has been defined as 'an end state which may or may not be the intended effect of specified inputs, outputs or processes'.[4] An amusing but far from unusual example, where the outcome was certainly not the intended effect of a particular output, has been highlighted in an account of an elderly woman's experience of dental care:

> I went to have my dentures and paid about £65 basic. When I came home they were so bad, my son said, 'Mum, why haven't you got your teeth in?' They looked terrible, so I went back to the dentist and said I'm not happy. She said that there was nothing that you can do about it, now they're made....They went in the bin and I put my old ones back in.[5]

The output of the service was the new set of dentures produced following the processes and procedures involved for which the dentist would have received the relevant fee. The outcome was that they were put in the bin!

This example could be an extreme case but the fact that death is now described as 'negative hospital output' highlights both the extent and difficulties of attempts to determine exactly what health care services produce. We now have the situation where death rates are used to assess the relative performance of the quality of the service provided by hospitals[6] – which perhaps gives credence to the claim by Stalin that 'a single death is a tragedy, a million deaths is a statistic!'

In the hospital sector, outputs are measured in terms of finished consultant episodes (FCEs), as highlighted in Chapter 3, with one patient hospitalisation potentially comprising a number of outputs. In primary care, general practitioners' remuneration is partly dependent on how they measure up to a series of targets designed to reflect quality of service, but this also tends to be based on outputs rather than outcomes. A study undertaken by the Office of National Statistics (ONS) in the UK, referred to in Chapter 1, showed that outputs to patients in the NHS rose by 28% during the period 1995–2003. However, the real resources pumped into the NHS over this 8-year period rose by 32–39%, after allowing for inflation in pay and costs. The gap between outputs and inputs is accounted for by what was termed 'tumbling productivity'. The ONS estimated that this dropped by 3–8% since 1995, which meant that if the NHS was as efficient as it was in 1995, it could achieve the same results for patients in 2004/05 with a budget £6 billion lower (nearly 9%) than the actual. The study also suggested that after taking into account rising costs and wage bills, for every extra £100 spent on the NHS, there would only be a £35 real rise in outputs.[7] However, as already indicated, there is no guarantee that these outputs will constitute a positive outcome from the patient perspective.

The question that has to be asked first is: what constitutes an outcome? It was defined above as the end state, which may or may not be the intended effect of specified inputs, outputs or processes.[4] However, even with such a definition, there are a number of contradictory and anomalous situations that can emerge. For example, the aim of assisted fertility treatment would be to produce fertilised eggs, which may result in a number of pregnancies.[8,9] Conversely, in assessing the effectiveness of contraception, the aim is to avoid the pregnancies from occurring.[10,11] However, even here it is difficult to disentangle what may be regarded as the outputs and the outcomes. Some authors do not make such a distinction and use the terms interchangeably, but it is probably wise to work on the basis of the definitions above, and adopt the premise that outputs are the deliverables generated by the functioning of health care processes and procedures, and outcomes are the actual impacts, on the recipients and others, arising from the outputs of the health care services. This is taken from the modified systems model, which is an 'extremely useful framework for analysing and evaluating policy processes within health care systems'.[12,13]

Identifying outputs and outcomes

In Chapter 3 the process of costing health care provision involved the three stages of identification, measurement and valuation. The outputs and outcomes resulting from health care also need to be identified and wherever possible measured and valued. In identifying outputs and outcomes it is possible to categorise them as shown in Box 4.1.

Box 4.1 Types of Outputs and Outcomes

Disease-specific/clinical effects	Specific outputs and outcomes resulting from health care interventions and services, such as reduction in cholesterol levels, improvements in symptom control, reduction in pain levels, return to normal functioning, successfully treated cases, number of at-risk patients identified.
Mortality and survival	Changes in life expectancy that may result from interventions and service provision and be expressed as life-years saved and lives saved.
Utility effects	Instruments that generate 'common currencies' to enable the health status of patients to be compared across all health care interventions, for example, healthy days and quality-adjusted life years (QALYs).
Economic effects	Resources released for other purposes as a result of interventions and services, translation of health benefits into monetary perspective.

Robert Macnamara is reported to have said that we must stop making what is measurable important and find ways to make the important measurable. The same publication also refers to a comment by Gertrude Stein, who said that for a difference to be a difference it has to make a difference. The book authors rightly argue that 'there is need to think differently, and realise that what has been measured in clinical trials, or what clinicians regard as outcome(s) may not be what patients perceive as outcome(s), nor what managers may want to use as outcome(s)'.[14] This is especially the case when attempting to assess the economic implications arising from particular interventions. It is often the case that clinical studies are powered to demonstrate a difference in effect, for example peak flow in asthma, but the impact on resources is often one of the secondary end points and there is no statistical difference because of the limited sample size. Similarly, individual studies are usually underpowered in measuring the extent of adverse events, but when systematic reviews are undertaken, the extent of adverse events can be enormous,[15] and one that places a very different complexion on the actual outcomes emanating from health care interventions.

Disease-specific/clinical effects

The views expressed so far have been reiterated in a discussion relating to what is meant by phrases conventionally used: 'clinically important difference', 'clinically meaningful difference', 'minimal detectable change', 'minimal clinically important difference'.[16] In some disease areas there are standardised measures used to determine outcome(s), such as lung function tests in the diagnosis and management of patients with asthma, blood pressure in hypertension, bone mineral density in osteoporosis and the American College of Rheumatology (ACR) criteria in rheumatoid arthritis.

However, within other areas one has to rely on what may be termed interim or surrogate outcomes.[17] These are indicators of what may be the actual outcome(s) in the normal progression of events, but in attempting to assess the effectiveness of interventions, there is insufficient time to allow normal progression to take place. A number of examples are to be found in health promotion initiatives, where success has to be measured in terms of people who quit smoking, for example, rather than following up such people to assess their actual survival or avoidance of smoking-related illnesses.

In the case of chronic diseases, where the aims of treatment are often to delay progression into disability, the choice of outcome can prove to be extremely difficult and contentious. In the case of relapse-remitting multiple sclerosis, it is not sufficient to merely document the impact of new therapies on the number of relapses suffered by patients; it is also necessary to include the duration and severity of each relapse as well.

The development and use of validated instruments to identify and measure clinical and disease-specific outcomes have burgeoned in recent years.[18,19] An example is the Index of Complexity, Outcome and Need (ICON), which was developed in orthodontic treatment to quantify deviant occlusal aspects of a dental malocclusion, with clear cut-off points for treatment need and outcome with categories for severity and improvement. A score of at least 43 indicated a need for treatment and a successful outcome was defined by a score of at most 30.[20] However, development of such instruments is not without its problems and issues. In a study using ICON to assess the cost-effectiveness of orthodontic service provision, it was shown that 8% of patients did not need treatment and a further 2% had an ICON score corresponding to an acceptable outcome prior to treatment commencing.[21]

Mortality and survival

George Bernard Shaw is reputed to have said that 'death is the ultimate statistic – one out of one will die!' While it is certain that everyone of us will die, what is uncertain is when that event will occur. Life expectancy is therefore an important indicator of outcome in interventions and programmes that aim to affect survival rates. Changes in life expectancy since 1950 and what it is likely to be in 2020 were reported in Chapter 1, but these are overall rates and do not reflect the extent of variation due to illness, ethnic origin, employment status and so on. In Chapter 3, the differences between developed and developing countries in terms of the diseases that affect mortality and morbidity were highlighted. It is indeed an incongruous situation that one of the biggest health problems in the West is that of obesity, a consequence of which is reduced life expectancy by 9 years on average,[22] while malnutrition and its effects continue to afflict many hundreds of thousands of people in other parts of the world – a poignant reminder of what Galbraith has called 'the theory of social balance' in which he reflected on the 'curious unevenness of people's blessings'.[23]

However, attempts to assess the impact of health care provision on survival rates are often difficult to estimate with any degree of precision, and reliance is often placed on surrogate and interim indicators, which are then used in modelling to predict the probable effects on mortality and survival rates. Further discussion on the role of modelling is provided in Chapter 5.

Utility effects/health-related quality of life

The impact of health-related problems on people's QOL has become a fertile ground for investigation in many discipline areas and the assessment of health-related QOL has been a complementary product of such developments. Many health care interventions and services do not (directly) affect life expectancy, but have a major impact on the ability of recipients to function and undertake normal daily activities. However, such approaches are not without their inherent problems. For instance, it is difficult to compare the health-related QOL of an elderly person, whose lack of mobility has meant that she has been housebound for a period of time and who receives a service that restores some degree of mobility to enable her to go shopping and visit friends and family, with that of the swimmer, who cut her leg on a camera and finished last in her heat, after being one of the favourites for a medal in the Olympic Games. Health-related QOL embraces a range of dimensions relating to both a person's physical and mental capacities, which can provide an indication of the utility that a person derives from receipt of a service.

The utility resulting from treatment and other health-influencing activities can be combined with survival to generate the QALY, which embraces both quality and quantity of life and provides a common currency for measuring the health gain resulting from health care interventions.

Economic effects

The notion that health economics is only concerned with monetary aspects of health care, or what things cost, or that health economists would argue in favour of those interventions that resulted in their recipients' returning to work and contributing to economic prosperity and paying taxes, have long since disappeared (hopefully).

It is nonetheless important to consider all of the resource implications resulting from health care provision. It is unfortunate that budgets have, in many senses, got in the way of this type of approach. The fact that costs are incurred by one budget holder, but that the returns and benefits accrue to another budget holder, used to be a recipe for the service not being implemented. Fortunately there are signs of improvement in that. For example, prescribing decisions, intended to ensure that drug budgets were not exceeded, now need to be made within a wider context, since the administration of a relatively high-cost drug may well prevent even more expensive hospital admissions, thereby producing a net benefit in terms of the overall budget and patient outcomes.

It is not difficult to identify economic effects, such as limited resources that could be used elsewhere as a result of fewer hospitalisations, working days gained following laser surgery as opposed to conventional surgical techniques and people's preferences for treatment benefits expressed in terms of willingness-to-pay (WTP). It is in the measurement and valuation of these economic effects that the most contentious issues emerge, to which attention will be focused later.

Measuring outputs and outcomes

Disease-specific/clinical effects

The measurement of clinical outcomes varies between disease areas. For example, in those areas for which there are well-validated standardised measures, it is relatively straightforward to assess whether an improvement in a patient's condition has resulted from the intervention. However, in other areas, this process is not quite as simple. For example, 'pain is a personal experience, which makes it difficult to define and measure'.[24] While it may be difficult to be completely objective, it is possible to envisage a number of criteria against which to assess the effects of interventions and pain management programmes. Most analgesic studies use pain measurement scales based on categorical scales or visual analogue scales, while the use of *percentage of patients achieving at least 50% pain relief* is increasingly used as an indicator of efficacy.[24] In terms of chronic pain the determination of outcomes is more problematic given the multidimensional nature of the problem,[25,26] but even here, the use of functional capacity, degree of disability, pain-free days, return to work, health-related QOL measures have all been advocated as potential indicators of effect. Despite the alleged difficulties in measurement, the evidence base for the effectiveness of interventions and management strategies in both acute and chronic pain is large.[24] In addition, it is continuously being updated, incorporating potential new therapeutic areas, interventions and management programmes[27–29] and increasing in quality,[30] while league tables for the efficacy of treatments are being developed,[31] based on numbers needed to treat (NNTs).[32–34]

In the case of rheumatoid arthritis the most commonly used outcome measure is the ACR response criteria,[35,36] a composite measure of seven indices:

(1) Tender joint count
(2) Swollen joint count
(3) Global disease activity assessed by observer
(4) Global disease activity assessed by patient
(5) Patient assessment of pain
(6) Physical disability score (like health assessment questionnaire)
(7) Acute phase response (C-reactive protein (CRP) or ESR measurement)

The ACR 20 response is defined as a 20% improvement in the first two of these, plus a 20% improvement in any three of the remaining five items. This is not an easy outcome to reach, although ACR 50 and ACR 70 are also being used now, which are similar to the ACR 20 but at 50% and 70% improvements. These are very high hurdles of treatment efficacy and represent very significant clinical improvement.

However, the problem with such measures is that they are specific to the disease area and cannot be used to compare with interventions in other disease areas. Therefore, measures that enable comparisons to be made across disease areas are more useful to decision-makers, who have to decide where to allocate additional resources. Traditionally, the emphasis was on mortality and survival but in recent years there has been a burgeoning of other instruments developed to provide some sort of common currency.

Mortality and survival

The effect of interventions on life expectancy can be measured in different ways; for example, in terms of patients alive in both arms of a clinical trial[17] or as the relative risk or odds of mortality in a given period of time in those who receive the intervention compared with those who do not.[37] Caution has to be exercised in measuring the impact of interventions on life expectancy and survival due to the multiplicity of factors that can affect mortality – it is essential that clinical trials conform to the highest standards if bias and misinterpretation are not to occur, as a result of not controlling confounding factors. In addition, it is not necessarily a straightforward process to transfer information relating to relative risk or odds of mortality into information about life expectancy – it depends on the age, sex, ethnic origin and other characteristics of the person, since life expectancy in the absence of the intervention is also dependent on these factors.[37]

In Chapter 1 reference was made to the difference in costs associated with saving one life as a result of preventing railway accidents as compared with the cost of saving one life by preventing road traffic accidents. A study in the USA estimated the cost per life-year saved for nearly 600 interventions designed to reduce premature mortality. For example, while cervical screening every 3 years for women aged 65 years and above would generate cost savings, annual screening for women aged 20 years and above would cost $220 000.[38]

Such data and information are obviously extremely useful to helpdetermine where resources are most appropriately allocated, but a further problem with reliance on mortality and survival as indicators of outcome is that in many disease areas it is the impact on morbidity that is more significant. Chronic disease management aims to reduce and relieve the debilitating effects of disease progression and ensure that patients are able to maintain normal functioning as long as possible. Interventions are specifically designed for this purpose and they would not score very high on a scale measuring the impact on life-years or number of deaths. As a consequence, measures that attempt to assess a person's QOL, as well as the quantity, are more effective indicators of the outcomes resulting from health care interventions and services in the area of chronic diseases.

Utility effects/health-related quality of life

Following the pioneering work of Rachel Rosser *et al.* in the 1970s,[39–42] a number of approaches have been used to generate health-related QOL valuations, which have endeavoured to encompass these dimensions in order to produce a profile of the person's health (e.g. the SF-36,[43] the Sickness Impact Profile,[44] the Nottingham Health Profile[45]) or a score to represent the person's state of health on a continuum between 0 and 1 or between 0 and 100, where 0 represents the worst possible health state and 1 or 100 represents the best possible health state (e.g. the EQ-5D,[46,47] the Health Utilities Index (HUI)[48,49]).

Box 4.2 shows the five questions in the EQ-5D, while Box 4.3 displays the visual analogue scale, which can be used to derive utility scores used in QALY calculations. Other approaches to the latter are the *standard gamble* technique and the *time trade-off* technique, both described in more detail in other articles and textbooks.[17,50–52]

The *standard gamble* approach presents individuals with a choice between living the rest of their life in their current health state and gambling for a return to perfect health or suffering immediate death. The probability of winning the gamble (i.e. returning to perfect health) is changed until individuals have no preference between the choices. If, when the probability of returning to perfect health is 0.75 and the probability of death is 0.25, an individual opts to live the rest of his or her life in the current health state, the probability will be adjusted upwards (e.g. 0.8) until the individual finds it very difficult to choose between opting for an 80% chance of returning to perfect health, but with the 20% risk of immediate death, and opting for a continuation in the current health state. The utility score attached to the current health state would be, in this case, 0.8.

The *time trade-off* method asks individuals how many years of perfect health they would trade for their life expectancy in their current health state. An individual who is expected to live for 20 years in the current health state who opts for 15 years of perfect health as the alternative would therefore have a utility score of 15/20, that is, 0.75 for the current health state.

The EQ-5D questionnaire is a standardised, generic instrument for describing and valuing health.[47] The five dimensions of mobility, self-care, usual activities, pain or discomfort, and anxiety or depression are divided into three levels, as shown in Box 4.2. Combinations of these levels provide 243 possible

---

Box 4.2 EQ-5D

Please consider your state of health *today* and tick one box for each question.

Q.1: Your mobility...
- I have no problems in walking about.
- I have some problems in walking about.
- I am confined to bed.

Q.2: Your self-care...
- I have no problems with self-care.
- I have some problems with washing or dressing myself.
- I am unable to wash or dress myself.

Q.3: Your usual activities (e.g. work, study, housework, family or leisure activities)...
- I have no problems with performing my usual activities.
- I have some problems with performing my usual activities.
- I am unable to perform my usual activities.

Q.4: Pain/discomfort...
- I have no pain or discomfort.
- I have moderate pain or discomfort.
- I have extreme pain or discomfort.

Q.5: Anxiety/depression...
- I am not anxious or depressed.
- I am moderately anxious or depressed.
- I am extremely anxious or depressed.

health states into which respondents will be placed, based on their answers to the five questions. For example, if a respondent indicated that there were no problems walking about, no problems with washing or dressing self, some problems with performing usual activities, moderate pain and discomfort and extremely anxious or depressed, this would be categorised as health state 11223 and would generate a utility score of 0.255.[53] The visual analogue scale, shown in Box 4.3, asks respondents to rate their perception of their

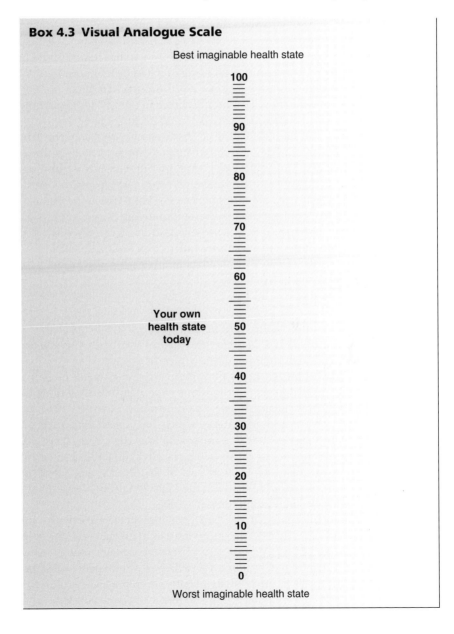

Box 4.3 Visual Analogue Scale

Best imaginable health state

100
90
80
70
60

**Your own
health state
today**

50
40
30
20
10
0

Worst imaginable health state

health in relation to the best imaginable health state (equivalent to 100) and the worst imaginable health state (equivalent to 0).

How good or bad is your health today?
To help people say how good or bad their health state is, we have drawn a scale (like a thermometer) on which the best state you can imagine is marked 100 and the worst state you can imagine is marked 0. We would like you to indicate on this scale how good or bad your own health is today, in your opinion. Please do this by drawing a line from the box below to whichever point on the scale indicates how good or bad your health is today.

The EQ-5D is now widely used in many countries and has been utilised in evaluating the effect of interventions on health-related QOL in a number of disease areas, and while it is not obligatory, NICE has suggested that the EQ-5D would 'appear to be the most appropriate choice in the UK' for generating QALYs.[54]

In North America the most widely used instrument is probably the HUI Mark 3 (HUI3).[48,49] In this system there are eight attributes: vision, hearing, speech, ambulation, dexterity, emotion, cognition and pain, with each having five or six levels and generating a total of 972 000 unique health states.

One of the most widely used measures of health-related QOL is the SF-36.[43] However, it does not generate a single score and therefore is unsuitable in its current format for deriving utility scores for QALYs. A SF-6D has been recently developed that uses an algorithm formed from the six dimensions of the SF-36,[55,56] but further work is needed before it becomes recognized as an alternative to the EQ-5D and HUI3.[57]

Economic effects
The process of converting health care benefits into monetary measures is fraught with difficulties. Two approaches have been used with varying degrees of success: the human capital and the preference-based.

The human capital approach relies on a monetary value being put on a human life, usually based on the earnings and potential future earnings of individuals. The approach obviously puts those members of society who are not productive at a distinct disadvantage, which has meant that such an approach is not often used in health care evaluations. However, there are numerous examples of monetary values being placed on disability and loss of life in other areas of public expenditure, while in determining levels of compensation, courts are required to assess the impact of death and disability on individuals and their families in monetary terms.

The preference-based approach assumes that individual preferences for particular health states or health care interventions (and their valuation of them) can be expressed by using the measuring rod of money[58] and by using what are known as contingent valuation techniques. Contingent valuation questions are used to elicit how much people are *willing to pay* for the benefits that are derived from a particular treatment or the health state into which they arrive as a result of the treatment.[59–63] This is the most common approach to measuring health care benefits in monetary terms,[58] but, as with all approaches, it is not without its critics and problems.[51,52,62] The advantages of contingent valuation in assigning a monetary value to health outcomes, in comparison to reliance on utility measures, have been highlighted, but the relative simplicity of such an approach 'may be a concern because respondents find it difficult, crass, reductionist or overtly materialistic'.[62] Examples of how this approach has been used to estimate the monetary benefits derived from health care interventions are discussed in the next section.

Another approach for eliciting the views of patients is that of discrete choice experiments, with evidence of the rationality and validity of the approach demonstrated.[64–74] These allow for the estimation of the relative importance of different aspects of care (including the cost), the trade-offs between these aspects and the total satisfaction or benefits respondents derive from health care services. It is also possible to incorporate a monetary valuation by the inclusion of cost among the attributes.

This approach is based on the premise that any service can be described by its characteristics (attributes), and the extent to which an individual values a service depends on the nature and levels of these characteristics. However, there are still problems in using such an approach,[75] but examples of its use are discussed in the next section.

Valuing outcomes and outcomes

Utility effects/health-related quality of life

The concept of QALYs has been discussed earlier in this chapter and that of DALYs as a measure of cost and burden of illness in Chapter 3. Despite their popularity, DALYs have been subjected to considerable discussion as to their suitability not only as a measure of disease burden but also as a vehicle for priority setting. It has been advocated that the case against DALYs is now strong enough to discard their use.[76] Therefore, the remainder of this section will focus on the concept of the QALY,[17,50–52,59,77,78] given its increasing importance in relation to health care decision-making, especially by authorities such as All Wales Medicines Strategy Group (AWMSG), NICE and the Scottish Medicines Consortium (SMC) (see Chapters 5 and 6 for further explanation of these bodies and their roles) in the UK and other similar bodies overseas.

The basic idea of a QALY is straightforward. It takes 1 year of perfect health to be worth 1, but regards 1 year of less than perfect health as less than 1. Thus an intervention that results in a patient living for an additional 4 years rather than dying within 1 year, but where the health-related QOL falls from 1 to 0.6, will generate 2 QALYs, as shown in Box 4.4.

With data relating to both health-related QOL and survival, it is possible to chart the impact of a health care intervention on an individual patient. One of the earliest applications of this technique, which has fostered subsequent debates about rationing and prioritisation in health care, was in the field of cardiac surgery and, in particular, coronary artery bypass grafting.[77]

Box 4.4 Derivation of QALYs

4 years extra life @ 0.6 (from health-related QOL valuation)   2.4
Less than 1 year @ reduced quality (1–0.6)   0.4
QALYs generated by the intervention   2.0

It is possible to compare the health profile of a patient receiving an intervention to that of a patient who does not receive it and plot their respective journeys through time. In Figure 4.1, a situation is displayed where treatment provides a consistently higher area under the QALY/time curve than with no treatment. In Figure 4.2, a situation is depicted where an intervention provides an initial superiority in health-related QOL, but because of adverse effects associated with the intervention the health-related QOL falls below that of the profile of the patient with no intervention. Given the difference in survival the issue then becomes one of 'deciding' between a longer survival time but at a reduced health-related QOL and a shorter survival time and a better health-related QOL.

It is no use pretending that QALYs are anything but a crude measurement of both survival and QOL as they currently stand. While they provide an indication of the benefits gained from a variety of medical procedures, in terms of QOL and survival for patients, they are far from perfect as a measure of outcome. For example, they suffer from a lack of sensitivity when comparing the efficacy of two competing but similar drugs and in the treatment of less severe health problems. Chronic diseases, where QOL is a major issue and survival less of an issue, are often difficult to accommodate in the QALY

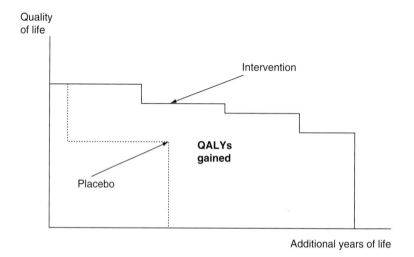

Figure 4.1 QALYs gained.

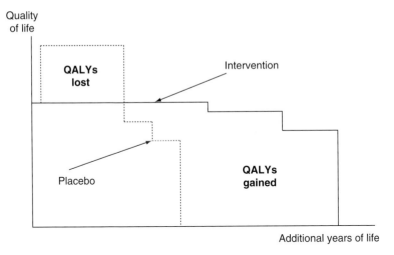

Figure 4.2 QALYs lost and gained.

context and there is a tendency to resort to the use of more specific measures of QOL. In health promotion and public health schemes, where the impact on health outcomes may not occur for many years, QALYs may be suboptimal, because the importance attached to each of the health dimensions is highly dependent on age, life context and life responsibilities.

Further criticisms relate to the inadequate weight attached to emotional and mental health problems, and the lack of consideration of the QOL of carers and other family members, while much debate surrounds who should be involved in placing values on health states. QALYs have also been criticised because there is an implication that some patients will be refused treatment, or not offered treatment for the sake of other patients. However, these choices would need to be made irrespective of whether QALYs or something similar existed, and even if the NHS were allocated a considerable increase in resources, it would still be necessary to make choices.

The use of QALYs in resource allocation decisions does mean that choices between patient groups competing for limited health care resources are made explicit, and, because they are recommended as a measure of health benefits resulting from health care interventions by NICE and other assessment bodies, their importance cannot be overemphasised.

The question that needs to be asked is: on what basis are choices and priorities being made? Are the decisions equally fair to all patient groups? Are there any patient groups who consistently receive less or poorer health care, or who consistently suffer poor health? As members of a society, doctors and nurses have a responsibility to the society as a whole and not only to individual patients, despite the fact that when faced with an ill patient it is painful to realise that treatment of this patient may be at the expense of another.

It should be the case that the choices made are efficient and humane, and not merely based on political pressures or the quest for technological advancement. There is a clear need for a constituency wider than the medical profession itself in assessing treatment priorities. To restrict decision-making to doctors, or for that matter administrators, is to allow the continuance of the current system of resource allocation where most resources go to those who shout the loudest or to those who pluck at the heartstrings the hardest. Widening the decision-making process is a move in the direction of ensuring a more humane system and the utilisation of QALYs (despite their limitations) is a means to include the outputs generated by the health care system in the process, thereby enabling decisions to be made that will maximise the benefits of health care provision for society.

In summing up this section it is worth remembering that there is no 'gold standard' or 'best' QOL measure, and it is probably best not to think in such terms. 'QOL is a subjective and fluid end point, so its measurement must include the patient's perspective and be sensitive to change over time. In addition to the important theoretical and empirical elements of QOL measurement, practical issues such as timing or administration ... are likely to provide obstacles to accurate measurement. ... It is important to be aware of the strengths and weaknesses of available measures when setting out to study QOL.'[79]

Economic effects

Willingness to pay
Participants in WTP studies are either asked what would be the maximum amount they would be prepared to pay or are presented with a series of WTP values and asked whether they would be prepared to pay that particular amount, as shown in Box 4.5.

Box 4.5 Willingness to Pay

At what level would you value a potentially effective treatment for your condition?
- I would value the treatment at *around £2* a month.
- I would value the treatment at *around £5* a month.
- I would value the treatment at *around £10* a month.
- I would value the treatment at *around £15* a month.
- I would value the treatment at *around £20* a month.
- I would value the treatment at *around £25* a month.
- I would value the treatment at *around £50* a month.
- I would value the treatment at *around £100* a month.
- I would value the treatment at *around £150* a month.

What would be the maximum amount you would be prepared to pay a month?

WTP was used in a study to determine the perceptions of diabetic patients of the priority of treating erectile dysfunction (ED) in comparison with treatments for other diabetic complications and relatively common medical conditions.[80] Consecutive patients attending diabetic clinics at two hospitals were invited to participate. Those who agreed were categorised into three groups: healthy diabetic men; impotent diabetic men; and impotent diabetic men not in a sexual relationship – while the partners of diabetic women attending the diabetes clinics (healthy males) formed a control group. As many as 243 questionnaires were returned.

The method of contingent valuation was used to measure people's WTP. Respondents were asked if they would be prepared to pay £2, £5, £10, £20 and £50 per month for the particular treatment and then asked to indicate the maximum amount per month that they would be prepared to pay. No indication of the costs of treatment was provided.

The amounts participants were willing to pay per month for a cure for each of the conditions are shown in Table 4.1. The control group was prepared to pay more for a cure for blindness than the other groups, while impotent diabetic men were prepared to pay more for a treatment for their condition than other groups. Given possible difference between the control group and other groups in income levels, an alternative approach was also employed, that is, the maximum amount each group would be prepared to pay per month for treatment for each of the conditions relative to the one that had the lowest WTP, which was mild indigestion. As shown in Table 4.2, the control group

Table 4.1 Maximum willingness to pay per month (£, mean ± SD).

Condition	Control group	Healthy diabetic men	Impotent diabetic men	Impotent diabetic men (not in sexual relationship)
Blindness	125.51 ± 126.43	62.97 ± 59.30	88.02 ± 153.50	33.22 ± 41.33
Foot ulcers	27.50 ± 43.23	28.23 ± 45.44	25.91 ± 31.50	20.98 ± 32.09
High blood cholesterol	19.27 ± 27.97	21.74 ± 41.13	15.62 ± 25.02	16.05 ± 27.61
High blood pressure	20.64 ± 25.69	29.16 ± 45.81	27.37 ± 65.41	17.67 ± 25.85
Impotence	38.98 ± 44.97	32.08 ± 50.95	50.54 ± 130.92	17.31 ± 24.37
Kidney disease	82.84 ± 80.70	56.33 ± 51.77	66.06 ± 99.19	41.76 ± 46.92
Migraine	20.51 ± 45.91	18.27 ± 40.60	14.33 ± 25.61	11.14 ± 24.80
Mild indigestion	6.29 ± 8.67	11.84 ± 35.39	7.52 ± 18.07	7.31 ± 17.98
Sleeping problems	15.46 ± 37.39	17.49 ± 38.16	13.49 ± 27.75	6.51 ± 8.63

Table 4.2 Valuations of each complaint expressed relative to valuation for indigestion.

Condition	Control group	Healthy diabetic men	Impotent diabetic men	Impotent diabetic men (not in sexual relationship)
Blindness	19.95	5.32	11.70	4.54
Foot ulcers	4.37	2.38	3.45	2.87
High cholesterol	3.06	1.84	2.08	2.20
High blood pressure	3.28	2.46	3.64	2.42
Impotence	6.20	2.71	6.72	2.37
Kidney disease	13.17	4.76	8.78	5.71
Migraine	3.26	1.54	1.91	1.52
Mild indigestion	1.00	1.00	1.00	1.00
Sleeping problems	2.46	1.48	1.79	0.89

would be prepared to pay nearly 20 times as much per month to cure blindness as to treat mild indigestion; they would be prepared to pay over 13 times as much per month to treat kidney disease and over 6 times as much to treat impotence. Diabetic impotent men would be prepared to pay nearly 7 times as much to treat impotence. The priority listing when all groups were included was blindness, followed by kidney disease and then impotence, and the same ordering applied when the control group was excluded.

Discrete choice experiments
Individuals are presented with choices of scenarios described in terms of characteristics and associated levels. For each choice they are asked to choose their preferred scenario. The responses are modelled within a benefit/satisfaction function, which provides information on whether or not the characteristics are important; the relative importance of the characteristics; the rate at which individuals are willing to trade between characteristics; and the overall benefit/satisfaction scores for the alternative scenarios.

In a study that aimed to establish which attributes of conservative treatments for non-metastatic prostrate cancer were most important, 129 men agreed to take part in the study and were presented with two treatment options, each containing a set of attributes at specific levels.[74] The attributes and levels are shown in Box 4.6.

In order to avoid overburdening the respondents the exercise was divided into two parts, with three attributes in the first part, three in the second and two that were included in both parts as shown in Box 4.7.

Box 4.6 Treatment Attributes and Levels Used in Main Discrete Choice Experiment (DCE)

Diarrhoea
• Absent
• Mild
• Moderate

Hot flushes
• Absent
• Mild
• Moderate

Breast swelling
• Absent
• Present

Loss of libido
• No
• Diminished

Maintaining erection
• No problems
• Occasional problems
• Unable

Lack of energy or 'pep'
• No problems
• Lacking

One-off out of pocket payment
• Range £0–400 (16 levels used)

Life expectancy
• Both options equal
• One option better by 2 months
• One option better by 4 months

Source: Sculpher et al.[74]

The study showed that men, having been told to assume a life expectancy of 5 years, were prepared to trade off life expectancy in return for 0.5 months of having no hot flushes or having them to a mild degree rather than having moderate to mild hot flushes; 1.3 months of moving from loss of libido (present) to no loss of libido (absent); 1.8 months of having mild or no diarrhoea rather than moderate to mild diarrhoea; 1.8 months of having mild or no problems in maintaining an erection from moderate to mild problems (0.9 months for men aged > 70 years); 1.9 months of having no breast swelling as opposed to having the problem; and 3 months of having energy or pep as opposed to having none.[74]

Box 4.7 Show Card Used in Discrete Choice Experiment (DCE)

	Option A	Option B
Part 1		
Sex drive or libido	Diminished	Diminished
Ability to get or maintain erection	No problems	No problems
Physical energy	Lacking 'pep'	No problems
Treatment cost to you personally	£400	£275
Life expectancy	Option A better by 2 months	
Part 2		
Diarrhoea	Present, moderate	Absent
Hot flushes	Present but mild	Present but mild
Breast swelling or tenderness	Present	Present
Treatment cost to you personally	None	£150
Life expectancy	Option A better by 2 months	

Source: Sculpher *et al.*[74]

However, it should not be assumed that DCEs are without problems. A number of problem areas have been identified[75]:

(1) Before being able to counter the use of DCEs in informing policies, it has to be made clear as to 'whose preferences about what are relevant to which policies'.

(2) There are concerns over psychological issues relating to the meaningfulness of the information generated.

(3) There are technical concerns due to the relatively small number of scenarios presented to respondents compared to the number of possible scenarios available from all combinations of attributes and levels.

(4) Can findings from DCEs be generalised to other situations? The authors argue that caution and circumspection should be exercised towards this technique at present.[75]

Other outcomes

The distinction between outputs and outcomes has been a theme throughout this chapter. What is also evident is that the provision of health care involves a series of processes, each of which has its own particular set of outputs and outcomes. For example, the patient episode is used as the 'unit of account' for measuring hospital activity but each episode can also be judged in relation to the quality of the care provided and the degree of patient satisfaction with the care provided and received. The quality of care provided can be measured in relation to predetermined standards, with incentives available for practitioners when quality standards are achieved, as in the Quality and Outcomes Framework of the GMS contract.[81] However, the problem is that this may result in the practice of ensuring that targets are met, which may not necessarily result in health gain being maximised in the community.

Patient satisfaction is another aspect that has been added to the array of measures and components associated with the effectiveness of health care provision. While it is apparent that the level of a patient's satisfaction is in many senses dependent on his or her expectations of the care process, there are three interrelated aspects of care that can affect the patient's experience: 'the clinical outcome, the physical environment in which care is received and the interpersonal relationships of care, namely how patients are treated by the carers.'[2] Patient satisfaction surveys remain the staple method for seeking the opinions of patients and ex-patients on a hospital's 'performance'.[82] Yet their construction is often the work of persons other than patients themselves. For example, an examination of many patient satisfaction questionnaires revealed a mix of poorly constructed questions, excessive number of items and little opportunity to attach ratings or scores to various aspects of the patient's experience, which adopted – in both research and ideological terms – an unethical inclination towards professional and/or managerial bias.[13]

Unintended outcomes

The costs associated with adverse events and other factors that inflate the costs of health care provision were discussed in detail in Chapter 3. While the case of Harold Shipman was, fortunately, a rare example of a health care professional who set out to deliberately cause harm to his patients, the incidence of errors, system deficiencies and other factors that compromise patient safety are receiving increased attention from politicians and policy-makers. For example, the initiatives to secure improvements in the rates of hospital-acquired infection are designed to reduce the financial burden resulting from such a problem, estimated to be nearly £1 billion per year in England,[83] the 'waste' of limited health care resources – beds occupied by patients who would have been discharged if it were not for them becoming infected and the loss of life in 5000 cases.[84]

The safety record of health care providers has been compared with that of the airline industry and found wanting.[85] It was estimated that it would be necessary to fly continuously for 20 000 years to have a 50% chance of an accident causing injury in an aeroplane. In medicine, by contrast, injuries from adverse events (from medical care itself) were found in 3.7% of hospital admissions in New York State hospitals, of which over half were preventable and about 14% fatal,[86] while in another study, serious or potentially serious medication errors were found in the care of 6.7 out of every 100 patients.[87]

If the risks of errors leading to serious injury or death were presented to aircraft passengers, the likelihood is that many would not choose to fly![85] Many other examples abound in the media of situations where patient safety has been compromised due to errors in the system, such as the tragic case of a patient who was due to leave hospital after successful treatment for leukaemia but died after contracting legionnaires' disease from a dirty shower on his ward.[88]

While the UK Government has committed itself to reducing by 40% the number of serious errors in the use of prescribed drugs, and has established the National Patient Safety Agency (NPSA)[89] to collect, collate, review and analyse error reports in order to accomplish this aim, the questions of how much we are prepared to pay to reduce risk, what risks we are prepared to accept and what outcomes are important still remain.

In conclusion, it is worth reiterating a statement made at the end of a conference, 'Measuring the outcomes of medical care', held in September 1989 organised by the Royal College of Physicians and the King's Fund Centre for Health Services Development. The final speaker, Anthony Clare – Clinical Professor of Psychiatry, Trinity College Dublin, and Medical Director, St Patrick's Hospital, Dublin – concluded the day's proceedings by stating:

> The assessment of outcome is too important to be left to clinicians, and certainly too subtle to be left to health economists, administrators and epidemiologists. Indeed, as this conference made clear, it cannot be left to any one group because it affects us all – politicians, professionals and the public.[90]

References

1 Marinker M, Blenkinsopp A, Bond C *et al.* (eds). *From compliance to concordance: achieving shared goals in medicine taking.* London: Royal Pharmaceutical Society of Great Britain, 1997.

2 Gillisen A. Managing asthma in the real world. *Int J Clin Pract* 2004; 58: 592–603.

3 Muir Gray JA. *Evidence-based healthcare.* Edinburgh: Churchill Livingstone, 1997.

4 Phillips CJ, Palfrey CF, Thomas P. *Evaluating health and social care.* Basingstoke: Macmillan, 1994.

5 Audit Commission. *Primary dental services in England and Wales.* London: Audit Commission, 2002.

6 Jacobson B, Midell J, McKee M. Hospital mortality league tables. *BMJ* 2003; 326: 777–78.

7 Office of National Statistics. *Public service productivity: health.* Paper 1. *http://www. statistics.gov.uk/cci/article.asp?id=987* (accessed 20 October 2004)

8 Garceau L, Henderson J, Davis LJ *et al.* Economic implications of assisted reproductive techniques: a systematic review. *Hum Reprod* 2002; 17: 3090–109.

9 Lloyd A, Kennedy R, Hutchinson J *et al.* Economic evaluation of highly purified menotropin compard with recombinant follicle-stimulating hormone in assisted reproduction. *Fert Steril* 2003; 80: 1108–13.

10 Phillips CJ. An economic review of long-term reversible contraceptives with particular reference to Implanon. *Pharmacoeconomics* 2000; 17: 209–21.

11 Varney SJ, Guest JF. Relative cost effectiveness of Depo-Provera, Implanon, and Mirena in reversible long-term hormonal contraception in the UK. *Pharmacoeconomics* 2004; 22: 1141–51.

12 Thomas P. Decision making and the management of change in the NHS. *Health Serv Manag* 1988; June: 29.

13 Palfrey C, Thomas P, Phillips CJ. *Effective health care management: an evaluative approach.* Oxford: Blackwell, 2004.

14 Moore A, Edwards J, Barden J *et al. Bandolier's little book of pain.* Oxford: Oxford University Press, 2003.

15 Tramer MR, Moore RA, Reynolds DJ *et al.* Quantitative estimation of rare adverse events which follow a biological progression: a new model applied to chronic NSAID use. *Pain* 2000; 85: 169–82.

16 McQuay HJ, Barden J, Moore RA. Clinically important changes: what's important and whose change is it anyway? *J Pain Symptom Manag* 2003; 25: 395–96.

17 Kobelt G. *Health economics: an introduction to economic evaluation.* London: Office of Health Economics, 2002.

18 Bowling A. *Measuring health: a review of quality-of-life measurement scales.* Buckingham: Open University Press, 1997.

19 Bowling A. *Measuring disease: a review of disease-specific quality of life measurement scales.* Buckingham: Open University Press, 2001.

20 Daniels C, Richmond S. The development of the index of complexity, outcome and need (ICON). *J Orthod* 2000; 27: 149–62.

21 Richmond S, Dunston F, Phillips CJ *et al.* Measuring the cost, effectiveness and cost-effectiveness of orthodontic care. *World J Orthod* 2005; 6.

22 Wanless D. *Securing good health for the whole population.* HM Treasury, 2004. *http:// www.hm-treasury.gov.uk./media/E43/27/Wanless04_summary.pdf* (accessed 12 January 2004)

23 Galbraith JK. *The affluent society.* Harmondsworth: Penguin, 1970.

24 McQuay HJ, Moore RA. *An evidence-based resource for pain relief.* Oxford University Press: Oxford, 1998.

25 Williams AC de C. Outcome assessment in chronic non-cancer pain treatment. *Acta Anaesthesiol Scand* 2001; 45: 1076–79.

26 Thomsen AB, Sørensen J, Sjøgren P *et al.* Economic evaluation of multidisciplinary pain management in chronic pain patients: a qualitative systematic review. *J Pain Symptom Manag* 2001; 22: 688–98.

27 Campbell FA, Tramèr MR, Carroll *et al.* Are cannabinoids an effective and safe treatment option in the management of pain? A qualitative systematic review. *BMJ* 2001; 323: 1–6.

28 Buchbinder R, Jolley D, Wyatt M. Population-based intervention to change back pain beliefs and disability: three part evaluation. *BMJ* 2001; 322: 1516–20.

29 Guzmán J, Esmail R, Karjalainen K *et al.* Multidisciplinary rehabilitation for chronic low back pain: systematic review. *BMJ* 2001; 322: 1511–16.

30 Moore RA. Pain and systematic reviews. *Acta Anaesthesiol Scand* 2001; 45: 1136–39.

31 Bandolier. The Oxford League Table of Analgesics in Acute Pain. *http://www.jr2.ox. ac.uk/Bandolier/booth/painpag/Acutrev/Analgesics/Leagtab.html* (accessed 20 May 2005)

32 Cook RJ, Sackett DL. The number needed to treat: a clinically useful measure of treatment effect. *BMJ* 1995; 310: 452–54.

33 Laupacis A, Sackett DL, Roberts RS. An assessment of clinically useful measures of the consequences of treatment. *N Engl J Med* 1994; 318: 1728–33.

34 McQuay HJ, Moore RA. Using numerical results from systematic reviews in clinical practice. *Ann Intern Med* 1997; 126: 712–20.

35 MacGregor AJ. Classification criteria for rheumatoid arthritis. *Baillieres Clin Rheumatol* 1995; 9: 287–304.

36 Arnett FC, Edworthy SM, Bloch DA *et al*. The American Rheumatism Association 1987 revised criteria for the classification of rheumatoid arthritis. *Arthritis Rheum* 1988; 31: 315–24.

37 Petitti D. *Meta-analysis, decision analysis and cost-effectiveness analysis*. New York: Oxford University Press, 2002.

38 Tengs TO, Adams ME, Pliskin JS *et al*. Five-hundred life-saving interventions and their cost-effectiveness. *Risk Analys* 1995; 15: 369–90.

39 Rosser R. From health indicators to quality adjusted life years: technical and ethical issues, in Hopkins A, Costain D (eds). *Measuring the outcomes of medical care*. London: Royal College of Physicians of London, 1990.

40 Rosser RM, Watts VC. The measurement of illness. *J Oper Res* 1978; 29: 529–40.

41 Rosser RM, Watts VC. The measurement of hospital output. *Int J Epidemiol* 1972; 1: 361–68.

42 Rosser RM, Kind P. A scale of valuations of states of illness: is there a social consensus? *Int J Epidemiol* 1978; 7: 347–58.

43 Ware JE, Donald C. The MOS 36-item short-form health survey (SF-36) conceptual framework and item selection. *Med Care* 1992; 30: 473–81.

44 Bergner M, Bobbitt RA, Carter B. The sickness impact profile: development and final testing of a health status measure. *Med Care* 1981; 19: 787–805.

45 Hunt SM, McEwen J, McKenna SP. Perceived health: age and sex comparisons in a community. *J Epidemiol Commun Med* 1984; 38: 156–60.

46 Brooks R. EuroQol: the current state of play. *Health Policy* 1996; 37: 53–72.

47 EuroQol Group. EuroQol: a new facility for the measurement of health-related quality of life. *Health Policy* 1990; 16: 199–208.

48 Feeny D, Furlong W, Boyle M *et al*. Multi-attribute health status classification systems: health utilities index. *Pharmacoeconomics* 1995; 7: 490–502.

49 Torrance GW, Furlong W, Feeny D *et al*. Multi-attribute preference functions. *Pharmacoeconomics* 1995; 7: 503–20.

50 Drummond MF, O'Brien B, Stoddart GL *et al*. *Methods for the economic evaluation of health care programmes*. Oxford: Oxford Medical Publications, 1997.

51 Jefferson T, Demicheli V, Mugford M. *Elementary economic evaluation in health care*. London: BMJ Books, 2000.

52 Dolan P. Output measures and valuation in health, in Drummond MF, McGuire A (eds). *Economic evaluation in health care: merging theory with practice*. Oxford: Oxford University Press and Office for Health Economics, 2001.

53 Dolan P, Gudex C, Kind P *et al*. *A social tariff for EuroQol: results from a UK general population survey*. York: Centre for Health Economics, University of York, 1995: Discussion Paper No. 138.

54 NICE. Guide to the Methods of Technology Appraisal, April 2004. *http://www. nice.org.uk/pdf/TAP_Methods.pdf* (accessed 22 December 2004)

55 Brazier J, Usherwood T, Harper R *et al*. Deriving a preference-based single index from the UK SF-36 health survey. *J CLin Epidemiol* 1998; 51: 1115–28.

56 Brazier J, Roberts J, Deverill M. The estimation of a preference-based measure of health from the SF-36. *J Health Econ* 2002; 21: 271–92.

57 O'Brien BJ, Spath M, Blackhouse G *et al*. A view from the bridge: agreement between the SF-6D utility algorithm and the Health Utilities Index. *Health Econ* 2003; 12: 975–81.

58 Mitton G, Donaldson C. *Priority setting tool kit: a guide to the use of economics in healthcare decision making*. London, BMJ Books, 2004.

59 Johannesson M. *Theory and methods of economic evaluation of health care*. Dordrecht: Kluwer Academic Publishers, 1996.

60 Johannesson M, Jönsson B. Economic evaluation in health care: is there a role for cost-benefit analysis? *Health Policy* 1991; 17: 1–23.

61 Olsen JA, Donaldson C. Helicopters, hips and hearts: using willingness to pay to set priorities for public sector health care programmes. *Soc Sci Med* 1998; 46: 1–12.

62 Bayoumi AM. The measurement of contingent valuation for health economics. *Pharmacoeconomics* 2004; 22: 691–700.

63 O'Brien B, Gafni A. When do the 'dollars' make sense? Toward a conceptual framework for contingent valuation studies in health care. *Med Decis Making* 1996; 16: 288–99.

64 Ryan M, Farrar S. Using conjoint analysis to elicit preferences for health care. *BMJ* 2000; 320: 1530–33.

65 Bryan S, Buxton M, Sheldon R *et al*. Magnetic resonance imaging for the investigation of knee injuries: an investigation of preference. *Health Econ* 1998; 7: 595–600.

66 Propper C. Contingent valuation of time spent on NHS waiting list. *Econ J* 1991; 100: 193–99.

67 Ratcliffe J, Buxton M. Patients' preferences regarding the process and outcomes of life-saving technology: an application of conjoint analysis to liver transplantation. *Int J Technol Assess Health Care* 1999; 15: 340–51.

68 Ryan M. Using conjoint analysis to go beyond health outcomes: an application to in vitro fertilisation. *Soc Sci Med* 1999; 8: 535–46.

69 Van der Pol M, Cairns J. Establishing preferences for blood transfusion support: an application of conjoint analysis. *J Health Services Res Manag* 1998; 3: 70–76.

70 Ryan M, McIntosh E, Shackley P. Using conjoint analysis to assess consumer preferences in primary care: an application to the patient health card. *Health Expect* 1998; 1: 117–29.

71 Farrar S, Ryan M, Ross D *et al*. Using discrete choice modelling in priority setting: an application to clinical service developments. *Soc Sci Med* 2000; 50: 63–75.

72 Ryan M, Bate A, Eastmond CJ *et al*. Use of discrete choice experiments to elicit preferences. *Q Health Care* 2001; 10(Suppl 1): i55–i60.

73 Van der Pol M, Cairns J. Estimating time preferences for health using discrete choice experiments. *Soc Sci Med* 2001; 52: 1459–70.

74 Sculpher M, Bryan S, Fry P *et al*. Patients' preferences for the management of non-metastatic prostrate cancer: discrete choice experiment. *BMJ* 2004: doi:10.1136/bmj.37972.497234.44 (published 29 January 2004).

75 Bryan S, Dolan P. Discrete choice experiments in health economics: for better or for worse? *Eur J Health Econ* 2004; 5: 199–202.

76 Lyttkens CH. Time to disable DALYs? On the use of disability-adjusted life years in health policy. *Eur J Health Econ* 2003; 4: 195–202.

77 Williams A. Economics of coronary artery bypass grafting. *BMJ* 1985; 291: 326–29.

78 Phillips CJ, Thompson G. *What is a QALY?* London: Hayward Medical Communications, 1998. *http://www.jr2.ox.ac.uk/bandolier/painres/download/whatis/QALY.pdf* (accessed 20 May 2005)

79 Erickson P, Taeuber RC, Scott J *et al.* Operational aspects of quality-of-life assessment: choosing the right instrument. *Pharmacoeconomics* 1995; 7: 39–48.

80 Rance JY, Davies S, Phillips CJ *et al.* How much of a priority is treating erectile dysfunction? A study of patients' perceptions. *Diab Med* 2003; 20: 205–209.

81 Department of Health. *Delivering investment in general practice: implementing the new GMS contract. http://www.dh.gov.uk/assetRoot/04/07/02/31/04070231/pdf* (accessed 16 January 2005)

82 Fitzpatrick R. Measurement of patient satisfaction, in Hopkins A, Costain D (eds). *Measuring the outcomes of medical care.* London: Royal College of Physicians of London, 1990.

83 Plowman R, Graves N, Griffin M *et al. Socio-economic burden of hospital acquired infection.* London: Public Health Laboratory Service, 2000.

84 National Audit Office. *Improving patient care by reducing the risk of hospital acquired infection: a progress report.* London: Report by the Comptroller and Auditor General HC876, July 2004.

85 Berwick DM, Leape LL. Reducing errors in medicine. *BMJ* 1999; 319: 136–37.

86 Brennan TA, Leape LL, Laird NM *et al.* Incidence of adverse events and negligence in hospitalized patients: results of the Harvard Medical Practice Study I. *N Engl J Med* 1991; 324: 370–76.

87 Bates DW, Cullen D, Laird N *et al.* Incidence of adverse drug events and potential adverse drug events: implications for prevention. *JAMA* 1995; 274: 29–34.

88 Lister S. Hospital shower kills cured patient. *The Times* 22 October 2004.

89 Department of Health. *Building a safer NHS for patients: improving medication safety. http://www.dh.gov.uk/assetRoot/04/08/49/61/04084961.pdf* (accessed 21 January 2005)

90 Clare AW. Some conclusions, in Hopkins A, Costain D (eds). *Measuring the outcomes of medical care.* London: Royal College of Physicians of London, 1990.

CHAPTER 5

Evaluating health care interventions from an economic perspective

Chapters 3 and 4 aimed to explain the nature of costs in health care and the outputs and outcomes that result from health care interventions and services. The aim of this chapter is to draw these threads together, and consider both the costs of providing services and the benefits derived from such health care provision, in providing an overview of the processes of economic evaluation as applied to health care.

Health care professionals are fully aware of the pressures facing the health service and initiatives relating to cost-effective prescribing; for example, they have merely served to reinforce the notion that patients have to be treated and managed within the contexts of clinical governance, predetermined formularies, new contracts and their quality initiative schemes, plus the perennial budgetary constraints, which seem to intensify each year. So how can an awareness of economics help those who are charged with making decisions about whether to make available a new therapy or new service, or provide assistance for those trying to convince decision-makers of the relative merit and worth of their products, therapies, interventions, programmes and services?

The influence and 'authority' of agencies, such as NICE, SMC and AWMSG in the UK context, which assess the relative merits of products within a treatment area in terms of clinical effectiveness and cost-effectiveness, has served to increase the importance attached to economic evaluations of therapies, pro- grammes and services in health care provision. The websites of the agencies[1] provide access to their specific requirements, but there are certain aspects that are common to them all, and this chapter aims to discuss these issues. Further discussion of their roles and requirements is contained in Chapter 6.

Health economic evaluation determines the efficiency of a service or activity by comparison with an alternative or alternatives, which may include no service provision. The basic framework of health economic evaluation is shown in Figure 5.1. Economic evaluation has been defined as a 'comparative analysis of alternative courses of action in terms of their costs and

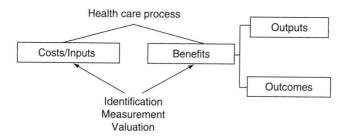

Figure 5.1 Economic evaluation framework.

consequences'.[2] From this definition it can be seen that evaluation involves some comparison between alternatives, which may include nothing, while the evaluation includes both the costs involved and the benefits that are derived from each of the alternatives.

Evaluating health care interventions from an economic perspective has been thoroughly covered in other books and articles[2-11] and interested readers are encouraged to access these sources. This chapter seeks to highlight the process, how it is utilised by decision-makers and agencies, and how health care professionals can appreciate and understand the relevance of its concepts in their practice. In addition, some of the difficulties and problems involved in the evaluation process are discussed, while it must be emphasised from the outset that the economic perspective is but one of the factors that comprise the decision-making process and is not the sole determinant of whether a therapy is introduced or a service provided.

In undertaking or assessing an economic evaluation of health care technologies or programmes, there are a number of requirements that must be dealt with or clearly stated. The first of these is to do with scope and context of the evaluation.

Scope and context of the evaluation

The scope and context of the evaluation must be clearly stated. This may be determined by the particular agency, which provides a clear specification of the treatment and therapeutic area. In other situations, such as in Scotland, where the onus is on the pharmaceutical company to submit a dossier of evidence to the Scottish Medicines Consortium as near as possible to the launch of a product, it must be made clear as to the role of the new therapy and where it fits in relation to existing products.

Perspective employed in the health economic evaluation

Since economic evaluations are used to assess the relative efficiency of alternative health care interventions, the perspective commonly taken is that of the health service. However, because of its foundations in welfare economics, it is preferable that economic evaluations should include the impact of an intervention on the welfare of the whole society, not just on the individuals or organisations directly involved, and adopt what is known as a social welfare perspective. One of the premises of economics is that individuals seek to maximise 'utility', and the aggregation of 'utility' across all individuals is known as social welfare, and it is assumed that governments, in taking decisions, aim to maximise social welfare. Thus, costs to the health service, to social services, to patients and their families and also to the rest of society, in the form of production losses etc., are included. However, in reality, narrower perspectives (e.g. the provider institution, the individual practitioner or professional organisation, the patient or patient group, the purchaser of health care, or third party payer) are usually employed, due to the difficulties involved in accessing relevant data or due to time constraints. Therefore, if the health economic evaluation is undertaken from the perspective of the health service, or from the perspective of the health service, social services and patients, it should be explicitly stated and the exclusion of items must be made clear, explained and discussed in terms of their likely influence on the final results.

The specification of well-defined alternative courses of action

The nature of the comparison being undertaken is vitally important, with a sound evidence base to support each claim and assumption. For example:
- Is a new product being compared with existing products and therapies?
- Is the comparison between a new technology and placebo?
- Is it a different dose or different route of administration?
- Does the product being awarded have a licence in an additional therapeutic area?

The relationship between the review of clinical effectiveness and review of cost-effectiveness must be readily apparent and provide a coherent argument for the clinical worth and value for money that the product seeks to represent.

In some cases, the choice of alternative is very clear, which could be no service or no intervention, or that which is currently held to be the most efficient method. Where this is not apparent, one way of identifying potential comparators is to consider the main objective of the intervention that is to be evaluated. Comparator programmes can be selected from other interventions that produce the same outcomes. The range of potential alternatives will be very large if the objective of the programme is broad and much smaller if the objective is narrow. For example, if the objective is to reduce smoking, specific alternatives aimed at preventing uptake or achieving quitting should be used. It may be possible to access published sources to obtain information on the costs and effectiveness of the alternatives, but it is important to consider whether studies undertaken in different contexts and settings and in different population groups can be legitimately used as comparators.

The nature of the comparison and the type of analysis to be undertaken

The type of benefit used informs the nature of the evaluation to be undertaken. Thus, *cost-effectiveness analysis* is used when outcomes are unidimensional and measured in terms of health effect, such as changes in blood pressure. When survival is the key measure of outcome, cost-effectiveness would assess the cost per life year gained from each of the alternatives with the lowest cost-effectiveness ratio indicating the best course of action.

When the outcomes generated by the alternatives are equal, it is possible to use *cost-minimisation analysis*, where the choice of the best alternative is made purely on the basis of cost. However, it has been argued that levels of uncertainty around both estimates of costs and outcomes call into question the relevance of cost minimisation.[12]

When outcomes are measured in terms of survival and QOL, such as QALYs, the technique used is that of *cost-utility analysis*. The beauty of cost-utility analysis is that it enables comparisons across different areas of health care – so that the cost per QALY of therapies designed to treat human immunodeficiency virus (HIV) and anti-immunodeficiency syndrome (AIDS) can be compared with those designed to treat people in advanced stages of cancer, as highlighted in Chapter 4. As the volume of cost-utility studies increased, a logical development was the construction of cost per QALY league tables,[13-15] an example of which is Table 5.1.

Table 5.1 Cost per QALY.

Intervention	Cost per QALY (£) 1990 prices
Cholesterol testing and diet therapy (all adults aged 40–69)	220
Neurosurgical intervention for head injury	240
GP advice to stop smoking	270
Neurosurgical intervention for subarachnoid haemorrhage	490
Antihypertensive treatment to prevent stroke (ages 45–64)	940
Pacemaker implantation	1 100
Hip replacement	1 180
Valve replacement for aortic stenosis	1 410
Cholesterol testing and treatment (all adults aged 40–69)	1 480
Docetaxel (as opposed to paclitaxel) in treatment of recurrent metastatic breast cancer	1 890

Continued

Table 5.1—*Continued*

Intervention	Cost per QALY (£) 1990 prices
CABG (left main-vessel disease, severe angina)	2 090
Kidney transplantation	4 710
Breast cancer screening	5 780
Heart transplantation	7 840
Donepezil, galantamine, rivastigmine for Alzheimer's disease (limited to those with mini-mental STTE score > 12)	8 700
Methylphenidate for attention deficit/hyperactivity disorder	9 600
Sibutramine for obesity	11 500
Cholesterol testing and treatment incrementally (all adults aged 25–39)	14 150
Infliximab for Crohn's disease	16 000
Home haemodialysis	17 260
Cox II inhibitors for OA and RA (for average-risk patients)	> 17 400
Etanercept and infliximab for RA	18 000
CABG (one-vessel disease, moderate angina)	18 830
Hospital haemodialysis	21 970
Zanamivir for influenza for all adults (for at-risk adults)	22 100 (11 900)
Riluzole for motor neurone disease	22 500
Laparoscopic surgery for inguinal hernia (compared with open surgery)	29 000
Beta-interferon and glatiramer acetate in MS	40 400
Erythropoietin treatment for anaemia in dialysis patients (assuming 10% reduction in mortality)	54 380
Addition of interferon-α2b to conventional treatment in newly diagnosed multiple myeloma	55 060
Neurosurgical intervention for malignant intracranial tumours	107 780
Erythropoietin treatment for anaemia in dialysis patients (assuming no increase in survival)	126 290

Note: Where range is specified, mid-point is used.
Source: Derived from Maynard,[13] Phillips and Thompson,[16] Towse *et al*.[17]

Cost per QALY league tables rank interventions by their average cost per QALY estimate and, when used in conjunction with a 'threshold', can help inform decisions as to how a limited amount of money should be spent to achieve the greatest health gain for the population by determining whether or not interventions represent value for money. A famous example of the approach was the Oregon experiment where the programme aimed to prioritise 1600 health problems on the basis of cost-utility ratios.[18,19]

However, despite attempts to improve the quality of the information contained within these tables and develop guidelines for their construction,[20,21] many problems with this approach have been identified.[4,22–24] QALY league tables have been accused of simplifying complex clinical situations. The studies underpinning the estimates may have been conducted in different settings and at different times, limiting their direct comparability. In addition, they often fail to do justice to the range of outcomes, brought about as a result of what may be termed health improvement. Use of QALYs as a single outcome measure for economic evaluation means that important health consequences are excluded and interventions that would not score particularly highly on the QALY scale can result in significant and profound effects.

For example, the impact of a baby born with Edwards syndrome (a chromosomal disorder that causes multiple malformations, severe mental impairment and a uniformly fatal outcome) on the patients in a local hospice was highlighted in an account given by the father of the child:

> Verity (*the mother*) sometimes used to visit the local hospice and take Christopher (*the baby*) round the wards. Here there were people who were dying and yet they were able to hold a baby who was also dying and in need of terminal palliative care. And somehow that shared experience between a baby who was dying and an adult who was dying was quite remarkable.[25]

The criticisms of QALYs emphasise the need for caution in their use in the decision-making process in relation to resource allocation. While cost-utility analysis may well be the 'most sophisticated method of economic evaluation so far developed to aid such decisions',[4] there remain many legitimate and important issues that illustrate the dangers of excessive reliance on economic evaluation, where 'this limited approach is followed by those who do not fully understand its basis and thus decisions are taken which neither reflect society's objectives nor its health beliefs'.[23]

The technique of *cost-benefit analysis* is used when the costs and outcomes are expressed in monetary terms; thus, as well as being able to make comparisons across all areas of health care, comparisons can also be made with schemes in education, transport and the environment. For example, it has been shown that contraceptive provision is an efficient use of public funds and secures considerable returns on investment.[26] The difficulty arises when trying to place a monetary value on the intangible benefits, where market prices do not exist. There are two main techniques that can be used here: willingness to pay and conjoint analysis (see Chapter 4).

When the outcomes are multidimensional – for example, changes in risk of cardiac events, myocardial infarctions avoided, strokes prevented, changes in blood pressure – the technique employed is that of *cost-consequences analysis*, where the outcomes are quantified and related to the costs for each of the alternative courses of action. This approach is beginning to find increasing support among health economists, as it does not restrict the outcomes generated from health care interventions and programmes to a single measure, such as QALY. It is easier to understand and enables decision-makers (on behalf of society) to impute their own specific, local values to these costs and consequences, and incorporate other aspects in the portfolio of information with which to inform the decision-making process.[23]

The identification, measurement and valuation of costs and benefits

The nature and categorisation of costs and benefits was highlighted in Chapters 3 and 4 respectively. The perspective employed in the valuation will determine the type of costs and the extent to which they are included: a narrow health service perspective will not include patients' costs, productivity costs and intangibles, whereas if a societal perspective were to be employed, all costs would need to be identified, and wherever possible measured and valued. In reality, this would not be possible, but the decision-maker needs to be informed how the analysis has dealt with costs and benefits that have not been specifically included in the calculations and in determining cost-effectiveness or cost benefit. This process is referred to as the sensitivity analysis, which will be discussed later.

How are costs and effects in the future dealt with?

The valuation of costs and benefits needs to reflect *when* costs are incurred and *when* benefits are realised. Individuals and societies are not indifferent to timing – preferring to delay costs as long as possible and to receive benefits as soon as possible. Most people prefer to delay costs as long as possible and receive benefits as soon as possible. Therefore, costs and benefits that occur today are valued more highly than those that will occur in the future, and the current value of any cost or benefit is lower the further in the future that it will arise. In order to allow for this, future costs and benefits are subjected to *discounting*.* In other words, all future costs and benefits are discounted to

---

* The approach is quite simple using the formula:

$$PV = K * ([1/(1 + r)^n])$$

where PV = present value, K = nominal value of the cost or benefit, r = discount rate and n = how many years in the future the cost or benefit will arise. If we expect to receive a benefit of £10 000 in 5 years' time, the present value, based on a discount rate of 5%, is equivalent to £7835.

bring them into line with what are termed present values. There is ongoing debate as to whether non-financial gains should be discounted, and the current recommendation from NICE is that costs and benefits are discounted at 3.5% and that the rate should be varied between 0% and 6% in the sensitivity analysis.[27]

Are incremental rather than absolute costs and benefits compared?

When a new treatment or service is being considered, it is unlikely that it will replace all existing and established therapies and services. Instead, some patients are switched while others will remain on existing treatments and services. In the context of clinical trials, new therapies are compared with placebo or exiting alternatives. The issue therefore is what additional benefits are gained from the additional costs of the new therapy? This approach is termed *incremental analysis,* where the difference in costs between the alternatives is divided by the difference in benefits. This provides a much more focused assessment of the impact of the new technology in context, rather than providing data relating to the total costs and benefits or the average cost and benefit generated by the new technology. The *incremental cost-effectiveness ratio* (ICER) – difference in costs divided by the difference in benefits – is used to address this issue. The ICER can be placed on a cost-effectiveness plane[28–30] as shown in Figure 5.2.

Interventions whose cost-effectiveness ratios are located in the north-west quadrant should not be provided because they result in a reduction in health effects and require additional resources. Those interventions that are located in the south-west quadrant result in a reduction in health effects but also

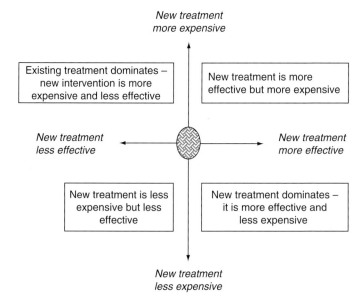

Figure 5.2 Cost-effectiveness plane.

result in resource savings. They are therefore often termed 'questionable'. Interventions with cost-effectiveness ratios in the south-east quadrant represent an improvement in health effects and at the same time provide additional financial resources to be spent elsewhere in order to improve the health of the community; they are termed dominant. But what about new interventions that are placed in the north-east quadrant – those that improve health effects but at a cost? Interventions with ICERs in the north-east quadrant require some consideration. They improve health but cost more than the alternative(s). The decision whether or not to choose them should be based on the level of additional resources available, or by viewing the ICER in the light of a specific acceptable threshold.[30] For example, interventions with cost/QALY ratios between £3000 and £20 000 were adjudged cost-effective when there was evidence of their effectiveness.[31]

More recently, there has been discussion as to whether NICE has a threshold value of £30 000 per QALY gained[32] – with interventions falling below this threshold value being approved and those falling above not being approved for use by the NHS. On the other hand, the claim that NICE has an absolute threshold has been strongly refuted, with judgements made on a case-by-case basis.[33]

Sensitivity analysis

The next issue is whether sensitivity analysis has been undertaken and how it has affected the conclusions. Economic evaluation is not an exact science and findings from such studies should be treated with caution. Uncertainty is a fact of life and no economic evaluation can do anything other than reach a conclusion on the basis of the best (most informed) assumptions possible. In undertaking economic evaluations there are four sources of potential uncertainty[34]:

- methodological changes arising from different approaches and methods employed;
- potential variation in the estimates of the parameters used in the evaluation;
- extrapolation from observed events over time or from intermediate to final health outcomes; and
- generalisability and transferability of results.

The wide variation in approaches and methods employed has led to the adoption of a reference case of core methods to be used when conducting economic evaluations.[27,35] For example, the NICE reference case is summarised in Box 5.1.

Box 5.1 NICE Reference Case	
Element	**Reference case**
Defining the decision problem	The scope developed by NICE for the appraisal
Comparator	Alternative therapies routinely used in the NHS
	Continued

Box 5.1 NICE Reference Case—*Continued*

Perspective on costs	National Health Service and Personal Social Services
Perspective on outcomes	All health effects on individuals
Type of economic evaluation	Cost-effectiveness analysis
Synthesis of evidence on outcomes	Based on systematic review
Measure of health benefits	QALYs
Description of health states for calculation of QALYs	Health states described using a standardised and validated generic instrument
Method of preference elicitation for health state valuation	Choice-based method, e.g. time trade-off, standard gamble (not rating scale)
Source of preference data	Representative sample of the public
Discount rate	An annual rate of 3.5% on both costs and health effects
Equity position	An additional QALY has the same weight regardless of the other characteristics of the individuals receiving the health benefit

Source: NICE.[27]

NICE does recognise that, in some instances, data required to present reference case results may not be available and that there may be important barriers to applying reference case methods. In such situations, NICE requires that submissions that are unable to meet the reference case requirements provide reasons that are clearly specified and justified, with the likely implications quantified. The NICE Appraisal Committee will then determine the weight it attaches to the results of such a non-reference case analysis.

It is also important to investigate how *sensitive* the findings of an evaluation are to changes in the assumptions used in the study and variations in the parameter estimates. Sensitivity analysis in such cases involves re-running the analysis with the assumptions changed and asking 'what if' type questions. 'One way' sensitivity analyses show the effects of varying each assumption separately. There are no rules regarding how much the original assumptions should be varied and a simple ±50% is often used. This allows caveats to be made about the original conclusion; for example, the conclusion that A is more cost-effective than B is highly sensitive to assumption X but not to assumptions Y and Z. It is also possible to vary the assumptions together – for example, to put a new intervention in the worst possible light. If on the basis of these collective 'worst case' assumptions the new intervention is still more cost-effective than the old, a change in policy is clearly indicated.

Another approach is to use *threshold analysis* where the variables are adjusted until the findings alter and the decision as to which therapy to adopt or reject is reversed. For example, to what extent do the costs of therapy A need to be increased to make therapy B cost-effective relative to A?

In recent years more sophisticated approaches have been employed to estimate the effect of uncertainty.[30,36] For instance, different methods have been used to establish the confidence intervals for estimates of ICERs, with the non-parametric technique of bootstrapping increasing in popularity.[30,37,38]

The bootstrapping method estimates the sampling distribution of the cost-effectiveness ratio through a large number of simulations, based on sampling with replacement from the original data. The cost and effects data from both intervention and control groups are sampled, and estimates of the cost and effect differential are obtained to generate the cost-effectiveness ratio. This process is repeated many times (usually 1000 times) and a vector of cost-effectiveness ratios obtained as shown in Figure 5.3.

However, when the individual costs and effects are not statistically significant, the bootstrap replications can straddle all four quadrants in the cost-effectiveness plane, and it is difficult to determine whether a new treatment is more cost-effective than current practice. One solution is to represent the bootstrap replications in the form of a cost-effectiveness acceptability curve,[30,36,39] as shown in Figure 5.4, in which the likelihood that the data are consistent with a true cost-effectiveness ratio falling below any given ceiling ratio, based on the observed size and variance of differences in the costs and effects in the trial, can be shown.

The problems associated with attempting to derive confidence intervals around the cost-effectiveness ratio have been overcome by the use of the net-benefit statistic,[36,40,41] where the ceiling ratio is brought into play by assigning the monetary value associated with it to determine the probability that the net benefit of the programme or intervention is greater than zero.

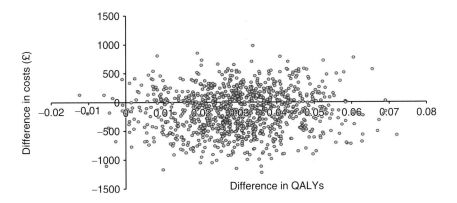

Figure 5.3 Results from bootstrapping.

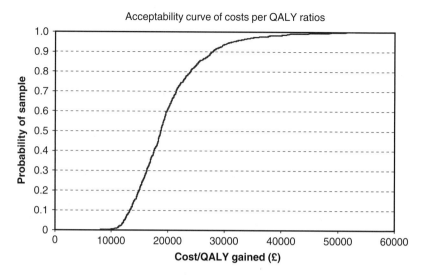

Figure 5.4 Cost-effectiveness acceptability curve.

The third potential area for uncertainty is associated with predicting from observational data or in extrapolating from intermediate outcomes to final health outcomes. Further discussion relating to sensitivity analysis within the context of modelling is provided later. However, the fourth area – that of generalisability and transferability – is now considered.

The relevance and applicability of the costs and outcomes

The relevance and applicability of costs and outcomes for the assessment agency is now analysed. For example, the relative cost-effectiveness of an intervention in the USA carries rather limited weight from English, Scottish or Welsh perspectives and it would be preferable if local costs and outcomes generated from relevant populations were utilised in a health economic evaluation. However, this may not always be possible and the onus lies with the evaluator to link the available evidence base to the situation and location over which the agency has jurisdiction. There are examples where a cost-effectiveness study undertaken in one country can be adapted and adjusted to reflect situations in other countries,[42–48] but there are many factors that can affect the findings when applied to specific countries. In a review, the unit costs associated with particular resources and measures of effectiveness were identified as the most frequently cited factors generating variability in economic results between locations.[49] While decision-analytic models have an important role to play in adapting the results between locations, evaluators need to ensure that sensitivity analysis reflects the range of confounding variables that exists and make explicit underlying assumptions used in studies which have crossed international and cultural boundaries.

Do the results indicate value for money?

The final component is to place the relative cost-effectiveness or cost benefit against accepted norms or benchmarks. This has been discussed in relation to cost per QALY league tables earlier, and there are examples of 'value for money thresholds' that have been advocated and used.[31,32,50,51] However, no decision-making agency has provided explicit threshold limits, and is very unlikely to do so. The question as to whether NICE has a threshold of around £30 000 per QALY gained has been referred to earlier, and while there are some who argue that this may be too high,[52] it is the case that they have approved interventions that exceed this amount and not approved interventions below this amount.[32] Therefore, the general consensus is that £30 000 per QALY gained represents the 'value for money' threshold in the UK at present.

However, in situations where it is not possible to produce QALY estimates, it is much more difficult to pronounce what constitutes acceptable value for money. One approach is to estimate the payback period – that is, the time in which the initial cost is likely to be repaid. This assumes that the effects can readily be translated into monetary effects. For example, the costs of contraception, the effects of discontinuations and the costs of treating adverse effects were compared with the cost implications of avoiding unwanted pregnancies, and it was shown that the monetary benefits resulting from the avoidance of unwanted pregnancies would repay the costs of contraception and its management within a period of months.[26] The limitations to such an approach are obvious but again it does provide information for decision-makers with which to assess the extent to which investment in health care services will reap rewards to society.

The role of modelling

Health economic techniques assist decision-makers to assess the most efficient way to utilise these scarce resources for the maximum benefit of society. In the evaluation of pharmaceutical interventions the most usual way to undertake economic assessments has been to piggyback clinical trials. However, the results of RCTs may have limited scope for generalisation to everyday patient management and may not represent the real world of clinical practice. In addition, the follow-up period within an RCT is often relatively short in relation to the natural progression of the disease. For example, while drug costs were the cheapest option when a relatively short-term perspective was employed, the cost of open or laparoscopic surgery was less than that of lifelong daily treatment with proton pump inhibitors (PPIs) or ranitidine for gastro-oesophageal reflux disease in Finland.[53]

The issue of lifetime long-term modelling is a contentious one in health economics, which has occupied many pages in books and articles.[42,54–58] However, the use of models 'is an important and necessary component of cost-effectiveness analysis'[58] and therefore cannot be neglected. However, the nature of chronic diseases necessitates that such perspectives are at least considered, so as to assess the future effects of early interventions. For example, treatment in the early stages of rheumatoid arthritis that effectively reduces long-term disability has the potential to save substantial costs to society.[59]

However, the nature of long-term is also conditioned by the nature of the disease and its progression. For example, a 20-year perspective is reasonable in relation to different hip prostheses,[60] as is a study that considered outcomes between 5 and 15 years in HIV interventions.[61] What may be somewhat surprising is a 10-year follow-up of patients with Alzheimer's[62] and a 5- and 10-year modelling process for women aged 60, 65, 70 and 75 for the treatment of postmenopausal symptoms.[63] However, these studies closely mirror the progression of the disease and the life expectancy of patients with such conditions. It therefore makes sense to adopt such time horizons. For other conditions, which occur earlier in life and yet which have consequences for the remainder of a person's life, it seems perfectly reasonable to utilise such time scales that reflect the duration of the disease across a person's whole life. The use of discounting ensures that benefits that accrue many years down the line are afforded an appropriate degree of diminution to enable present-day valuations to be employed.

Furthermore, the fact is that as a condition deteriorates, the resource consequences are likely to increase exponentially, and it is therefore important from an economic as well as a clinical point of view, to delay disease progression as much as possible.[46]

One fully recognises the potential tension between long-term benefits and short-term costs and their impact on budgets,[64] but as long as decision-makers are made aware of the issues and the need for possible trade-offs, the two approaches can live comfortably together.

Decision analysis

Decision-analysis models are used to simplify situations to a level that describes the essential consequences and complications of different options for decision-makers. Two types of decision-analysis models are generally used in health economic evaluations: decision-tree and Markov.

Decision-tree models incorporate the choices that have to be made in deciding between options in patient management strategies, for example, the probability of events occurring, and their costs, as a result of the options being chosen and the probability of final outcomes occurring together with their respective utilities (if appropriate) and costs. In decision-tree models,

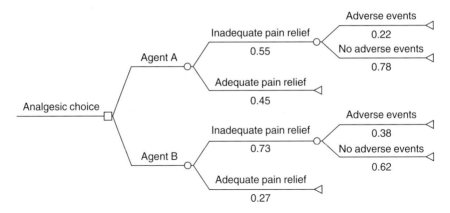

Figure 5.5 Decision tree for analgesic choice.

decisions are represented as squares (decision nodes) and the branches form the relevant options. Circles are used to represent chance nodes, which are the events and outcomes resulting from the decision. Due to the uncertainty surrounding these events and outcomes, probabilities are assigned to each of them – with the summation of all probabilities being equal to 1. The expected cost of each option is derived by multiplying the cost for each branch by the probability of that branch occurring and enabling the options to be compared in terms of their respective costs and outcomes. This is shown diagrammatically in Figure 5.5.

In Figure 5.5, the choice is between two analgesic agents, which have different levels of efficacy, safety and costs. The acquisition cost of Agent A is £350; it secures 50% reduction in pain at 6 h in 45% of patients with no adverse events recorded; and is associated with a 22% probability of any adverse event occurring in those for whom the agent is not effective. The acquisition cost of Agent B is £130; it secures 50% reduction in pain at 6 h in 27% of patients with no adverse events recorded; and is associated with a 38% probability of any adverse event occurring in those for whom the agent is not effective. The cost of treating an adverse event has been estimated at £500 on average.

The total cost of using Agent A in 100 patients is £41 050:

$[(100 \times 350) + (0.22 \times 0.55 \times 100 \times 500)]$

Cost per successfully treated patient for Agent A is £912 (41050/45).

The total cost of using Agent B in 100 patients is £26 870:

$[100 \times 130) + (0.38 \times 0.73 \times 100 \times 500)]$

Cost per successfully treated patient for Agent B is £995 (26870/27).

Decision-tree models are often too simplistic to describe situations where there are many alternative scenarios or in the case of chronic disease where the same decisions are constantly repeated over time. In such situations, Markov models are usually used. These are a particular type of decision analysis that allows for the transfer between different health states over a period of time. The structure of a Markov model is shown in Figure 5.6.

In a Markov model, the disease is categorised into a finite set of health states (referred to as Markov states), usually based on disease parameters, such as the severity of the disease, which are meaningful to clinicians and patients. Patients move between these health states over a clinically mean-ingful discrete period of time (e.g. 1 month, 1 year) according to a set of transition probabilities, which reflect disease progression and the effective-ness of interventions to reverse or reduce the extent of progression. These time periods, Markov cycles, must be relevant within the context of the specific disease – for example, weekly or monthly periods may be appropriate in a pain management programme, while for multiple sclerosis these periods may be too short. Transition probabilities are derived from evidence gathered from systematic reviews, clinical trials or epidemiological studies, while costs and utilities are attached to each particular Markov state to estimate the long-term costs and outcomes for patient cohorts who have the disease and are receiving relevant health care interventions.

In order for the Markov process to terminate, it must have at least one 'absorbing state', which patients cannot leave. This is usually death in most examples of Markov models, and the process continues until all patients have been absorbed by this particular state. The length of the Markov process and number of Markov cycles is therefore conditioned by the nature of the disease

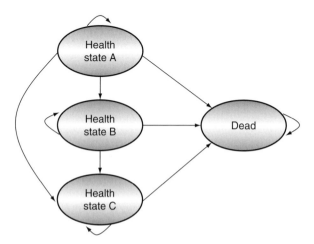

Figure 5.6 Markov model.

and its progression. What is important is that Markov models closely mirror the progression of the disease and the life expectancy of patients with particular conditions, and for some diseases, which are diagnosed early in life and yet which have consequences for the remainder of a person's life, the model needs to reflect such time scales in the number of cycles it contains.

There are a few notes of caution when interpreting studies based on modelling:

(1) The quality of the model is highly dependent on the quality of the clinical data used to furnish the model. The use of data from small-scale trials to derive a model of the cost-effectiveness of an intervention across a broad population spectrum should be treated with suspicion.

(2) The use of observational data in models is subject to considerable bias and different interpretations and should be regarded with a large element of circumspection.

(3) The problems associated with extrapolation from clinical trials imply that models based on such data are by default subject to those very problems, and the incorporation of this type of data into a model does nothing to reduce its deficiencies.

(4) The scope for manipulation with models is much greater than with RCTs, given the nature of inclusion and exclusion criteria in the latter, and therefore the need for a health warning on the interpretation of models cannot be overemphasised.

It may be that the term *cost-efficacy models* be used, rather than *cost-effectiveness models*, to describe models that have been developed and furnished with data from clinical trials of relatively short duration, in relation to the lifetime of a disease, and undertaken under conditions that do not always accurately portray everyday clinical practice.

The increased use of models and reliance on them for assessing cost-effectiveness have been accompanied by an increased awareness to ensure that variation and uncertainty in the model parameters are adequately dealt with. The use of probabilistic sensitivity analysis as a method for handling uncertainty in cost-effectiveness models[30,65] is increasingly becoming the norm, as it enables the production of cost-effectiveness acceptability curves to assist the decision-making process.

There is currently no 'gold standard' approach to modelling, but given the increasing importance and use of models in health economic evaluations and decisions relating to the adoption of new technologies, there is a need to ensure that best practice is employed and that the limitations of such approaches are clear and explicit in the reporting of such studies.[42,54–58,66]

Currently, modelling cannot be a substitute for obtaining reliable and prospective evidence but should be regarded as a complement for real-time evaluation,[66] which provides decision-makers with useful information to assess current and new therapies. It is important that their limitations be recognised,[58] but in order to enhance the quality and accuracy of models used

in health economic evaluations the following suggestions have been proposed[66]:
- Models should be designed and conducted using the best available practices
  according to the objectives of the study.
- The methodology employed ought to be explicitly and transparently
  reported, to enable comparability among all analyses.
- The software package used to construct the model should be referenced and
  a copy of the model should be made available to relevant agencies.
- Financial arrangements between sponsor and investigators/modellers
  should be explicit.

Issues in evaluating health care interventions from the economic perspective

The decision-making process in determining which services and treatments
should be provided is highly complex and involves a number of different,
often conflicting, factors. Health economic techniques can assist decision-
makers to utilise the information relating to the effectiveness and efficiency
of an intervention. They can also go some way in contributing to the commissioning process in determining health care priorities and in seeking to
ensure that the most efficient use is made of resources available within
limited health care budgets. However, the cost and time required to undertake full-blown economic evaluations render them unfeasible in the context
of many decisions.[67] It has also been argued that the assumptions underlying
the current methods fail to consider all society's health objectives and are too
complex for policymakers to use. In addition, 'by generating a pseudoscien-
tific aura around economic evaluation, they camouflage critical weaknesses
in current techniques'.[23] It is argued that the assumption that the aim of
decision-makers is to maximise health benefits to society from available
resources is highly questionable.

> Even aside from doubts over the existence of this mythical decision-
> maker with a clear set of objectives, the desire to maximise health seems
> to be largely the objective of economists rather than [of] society.[23]

It is unlikely that resource allocation decisions are solely based on the maximisation of health care benefits; if so, no resources would be allocated to
services provided for extremely rare conditions, with poor survival and QOL
outcomes. Rather decisions are based on many factors, of which the maximisation of health is but one alongside equity, need, access and so on.

In addition, attempts to restrict the benefits derived from health care
services into a single outcome measure also fail to do justice to the wide-
ranging impact that health care improvements can have on patients, their
families, their communities and society as a whole. Many of the recent
developments in economic evaluation in health care have been encapsulated

in the 'biggest bang per buck' philosophy, with the focus on the economics of health care and insufficient attention given to the other features of the determinants of health model.[68]

The emphasis on cost-effectiveness may also lead to overspending.[67] For example, therapies and treatments, which have been given the NICE stamp of approval, are recommended for use by the NHS and are expected to be made available within a 3–6-month period. While the introduction of such a therapy may not necessarily impose a significant additional burden on budgets per se, the aggregation of a number of therapies, all of which generate additional health benefits at relatively low cost, may well cause major financial problems for both providers and commissioners of health care services, and lead to a suboptimal allocation of resources as organisations, limited by the imposition of financial targets as well, are 'forced' into making cutbacks in other areas to finance the treatments approved by NICE.[69]

Another criticism levied at the door of NICE is that its focus on new technologies and relatively little attention devoted to existing and old technologies that 'may be redundant'[70] has led to inflationary pressure, while the emphasis on incremental cost-effectiveness ratios in the shape of cost per QALY ratios is 'not compatible with the most basic principle in economics of opportunity costs'.[71]

Chapter 6 further explores some of the issues involved in the utilisation of economic evaluation techniques by decision-makers and outlines other approaches that can assist decision-makers as they struggle to balance the competing claims made on limited resources by a variety of parties, each of whom have strong and worthy rationales to underpin their particular case.

References

1 NICE. http://www.nice.org.uk (accessed 22 December 2004); SMC. http://www.scottishmedicines.org (accessed 12 January 2005); AWMSG. http://www.wales.nhs.uk/awmsg (accessed 12 January 2005)

2 Drummond MF, O'Brien B, Stoddart GL *et al. Methods for the economic evaluation of health care programmes.* Oxford: Oxford Medical Publications, 1997.

3 Sloan F (ed). *Valuing health care: costs, benefits and effectiveness of pharmaceuticals and other medical technologies.* Cambridge: Cambridge University Press, 1996.

4 Jefferson T, Demicheli V, Mugford M. *Elementary economic evaluation in health care.* London: BMJ Books, 2000.

5 Kobelt G. *Health economics: an introduction to economic evaluation.* London: Office for Health Economics, 2002.

6 Johannesson M. *Theory and methods of economic evaluation of health care.* Dordrecht: Kluwer Academic Publishers, 1996.

7 McCrone PR. *Understanding health economics: a guide for health care decision makers.* London: Kogan Page, 1998.

8 McGuire A, Henderson J. *The economics of health care: an introductory text.* London: Routledge and Kegan Paul, 1987.

 9 Phillips CJ, Palfrey CF, Thomas P. *Evaluating health and social care.* Basingstoke, Macmillan, 1994.

10 Drummond MF, McGuire A (eds). *Economic evaluation in health care: merging theory with practice.* Oxford: Oxford University Press, 2001.

11 Petitti D. *Meta-analysis, decision analysis and cost-effectiveness analysis.* New York: Oxford University Press, 2002.

12 Briggs AH, O'Brien BJ. The death of cost-minimisation analysis? *Health Econ* 2001; 10: 179–84.

13 Maynard A. Developing the healthcare market. *Econ J* 1991; 101: 1277–86.

14 Williams A. Economics of coronary artery bypass grafting. *BMJ* 1985; 291: 326–29.

15 Laupacis A, Feeny D, Detsky AS *et al.* How attractive does a new technology have to be to warrant adoption and utilization? Tentative guidelines for using clinical and economic evaluations. *Can Med Assoc J* 1992; 146: 473–81.

16 Phillips CJ, Thompson G. What s a QALY? London: Hayward Medical Communications, 1998. *www.jr2.ox.ac.uk/bandolier/painter/download/what is/QALY.pdf*

17 Towse A, Pritchard C. Does NICE have a threshold? An external view, in Towse A, Pritchard C, Devlin N (eds). *Cost-effectiveness threshold: economic and ethical issues.* London: Office of Health Economics, 2003.

18 Blumstein JF. The Oregon experiment: the role of cost-benefit analysis in the allocation of Medicaid funds. *Soc Sci Med* 1997; 45: 545–54.

19 Brannigan M. Oregon's experiment. *Health Care Anal* 1993; 1: 15–32.

20 Mason JM, Drummond MF, Torrance GW. Some guidelines on the use of cost-effectiveness league tables. *BMJ* 1993; 306: 570–72.

21 Mason JM. Cost per QALY league tables: their use in pharmacoeconomic analysis. *Pharmacoeconomics* 1994; 5: 472–81.

22 Petrou S, Malek M, Davey P. The reliability of cost-utility estimates in cost per QALY league tables. *Pharmacoeconomics* 1993; 3: 345–53.

23 Coast J. Is economic evaluation in touch with society's health values? *BMJ* 2004; 329: 1233–36.

24 Gerard K, Mooney G. QALY league tables: handle with care. *Health Econ* 1993; 2: 59–64.

25 Wyatt J. *Matters of life and death: today's healthcare dilemmas in the light of the Christian faith.* Leicester: Inter-Varsity Press, 1998.

26 Phillips CJ. An economic review of long-term reversible contraceptives with particular reference to Implanon. *Pharmacoeconomics* 2000; 17: 209–21.

27 National Institute of Clinical Excellence. *www.nice.org.uk/pdf/TAP_Methods.pdf* (accessed 22 December 2004)

28 Anderson JP, Bush JW, Clen M, Dolenc P. Policy space areas and properties of benefit-cost/utility analysis. *J Am Med Assoc* 1986; 255: 794–95.

29 Black WC. The CE plane: a graphic representation of cost-effectiveness. *Med Decision-Making* 1990; 10: 212–14.

30 Briggs AH. Handling uncertainty in economic evaluation and presenting the results, in Drummond MF, McGuire A (eds). *Economic evaluation in health care: merging theory with practice.* Oxford: Oxford University Press, 2001.

31 Stevens A, Colin-Jones D, Gabbay J. Quick and clean: authoritative health technology assessment for local health care contracting. *Health Trends* 1995; 27: 37–42.

32 Towse A, Pritchard C. Does NICE have a threshold? An external view, in Towse A, Pritchard C, Devlin N (eds). *Cost-effectiveness thresholds: economic and ethical issues.* London: Office of Health Economics, 2003.

33 Rawlins MD, Culyer AJ. National Institute for Clinical Excellence and its value judgements. *BMJ* 2004; 329: 224–27.

34 Briggs A, Sculpher M, Buxton M. Uncertainty in the economic evaluation of healthcare technologies: the role of sensitivity analysis. *Health Econ* 1994; 3: 95–104.

35 Gold MR, Siegel JE, Russell LB *et al. Cost-effectiveness in health and medicine.* New York: Oxford University Press, 1996.

36 Glick HA, Briggs AH, Polsky D. Quantifying stochastic uncertainty and presenting results of cost-effectiveness analyses. *Expert Rev Pharmacoecon Outcomes Res* 2001; 1: 25–36.

37 Briggs AH, Wonderling DE, Mooney CZ. Pulling cost-effectiveness analysis up by its bootstraps: a non-parametric approach to confidence interval estimation. *Health Econ* 1997; 6: 327–40.

38 Briggs AH, Wonderling DE, Mooney CZ. Constructing confidence intervals for cost-effectiveness ratios: an evaluation of parametric and non-parametric techniques using Monte Carlo simulation. *Stat Med* 1999; 18: 3245–62.

39 Fenwick E, O'Brien BJ, Briggs A. Cost-effectiveness acceptability curves: facts, fallacies and frequently asked questions. *Health Econ* 2004; 13: 405–15.

40 Claxton K. The irrelevance of inference: a decision-making approach to the stochastic evaluation of healthcare technologies. *J Health Econ* 1999; 18: 341–64.

41 Stinnett AA, Mullahy J. Net benefits: a new framework for the analysis of uncertainty in cost-effectiveness analysis. *Med Decision-Making* 1998; 18: S65–S80.

42 Siebert U. When should decision-analytic modelling be used in the economic evaluation of health care? *Eur J Health Econ* 2003; 4: 143–50.

43 Stein K, Roesnberg W, Wong J. Cost effectiveness of combination therapy for hepatitis C: a decision analytic model. *Gut* 2002; 50: 253–58.

44 Wong JB, Poynard T, Ling MH *et al.* Cost-effectiveness of 24 or 48 weeks of interferon alpha-2b alone or with ribavirin as initial treatment of chronic hepatitis C: International Hepatitis Interventional Therapy Group. *Am J Gastroenterol* 2000; 95: 1524–30.

45 Siebert U, Sroczynski G, Rossol S *et al.* Cost effectiveness of peginterferon alpha-2b plus ribavirin versus interferon alpha-2b plus ribavirin for initial treatment of chronic hepatitis C. *Gut* 2003; 52: 425–32.

46 Miltenburger C, Kobelt G. Quality of life and cost of multiple sclerosis. *Clin Neurol Neurosurg* 2002; 104: 272–75.

47 Kobelt G, Lindgren P, Smala A *et al.* Costs and quality of life in multiple sclerosis: an observational study in Germany. *HEPAC* 2001; 2: 60–68.

48 Kobelt G, Lindgren P, Parkin D *et al. Costs and quality of life in multiple sclerosis: a cross-sectional observational study in the United Kingdom.* EFI Research Report No. 398. Stockholm: Stockholm School of Economics, 2000.

49 Sculpher MJ, Pang FS, Manca A *et al.* Generalisability in economic evaluation studies in healthcare: a review and case studies. *Health Tech Assess* 2004; 8: 49.

50 Johannesson M. The cost-effectiveness of hypertension treatment in Sweden. *Pharmacoeconomics* 1995; 7: 242–50.

51 Kuntz KM, Lee TH. Cost-effectiveness of accepted measures for intervention in coronary heart disease. *Coron Artery Dis* 1995; 6: 472–48.

52 Williams A. *What could be nicer than NICE?* London: Office of Health Economics, 2004.

53 Viljakka M, Nevalainen J, Isolauri J. Lifetime costs of surgical versus medical treatment of severe gastro-oesophageal reflux disease in Finland. *Scand J Gastroenterol* 1997; 32: 766–72.

54 Buxton MJ, Drummond MF, Van Hout BA *et al.* Modelling in economic evaluation: an unavoidable fact of life. *Health Econ* 1997; 6: 217–27.

55 Weinstein MC, Toy EL, Sandberg EA *et al.* Modelling for healthcare and other policy decisions: uses, roles and validity. *Value Health* 2001; 4: 348–61.

56 Sheldon TA. Problems of using modelling in the economic evaluation of healthcare. *Health Econ* 1996; 5: 1–11.

57 Rittenhouse B. *Uses of models in economic evaluations of medicines and other health technologies.* London: Office of Health Economics, 1996.

58 Kuntz KM, Weinstein MC. Modelling in economic evaluation, in Drummond MF, McGuire A (eds). *Economic evaluation in health care: merging theory with practice.* Oxford: Oxford University Press, 2001.

59 Pugner KM, Scott DI, Holmes JW *et al.* The costs of rheumatoid arthritis: an international long-term view. *Semin Arthritis Rheum* 2000; 29: 305–20.

60 Baxter K, Bevan G. An economic model to estimate the relative costs over 20 years of different hip prostheses. *J Epidemiol Commun Health* 1999; 53: 542–47.

61 Caro J, O'Brien JA, Migliaccio-Walle K, Raggio G. Economic analysis of initial HIV therapy. *Pharmacoeconomics* 2001; 19: 95–104.

62 McDonnell J, Redekop WK, van der Roer N *et al.* The cost of treatment of Alzheimer's disease in the Netherlands. *Pharmacoeconomics* 2001; 19: 379–90.

63 Coyle D, Cranney A, Lee KM *et al.* Cost effectiveness of nasal calcitonin in postmenopausal women. *Pharmacoeconomics* 2001; 19: 565–75.

64 Trueman P, Drummond M, Hutton J. Developing guidance for budget impact analysis. *Pharmacoeconomics* 2001; 19: 609–21.

65 Briggs AH. Handling uncertainty in cost-effectiveness models. *Pharmacoeconomics* 2000; 17: 479–500.

66 Soto J. Health economic evaluations using decision analytic modelling. *Int J Tech Assess Health Care* 2002; 18: 94–111.

67 Mitton G, Donaldson C. *Priority setting tool kit: a guide to the use of economics in healthcare decision making.* London, BMJ Books, 2004.

68 Evans RG, Stoddart GL. Producing health, consuming health care. *Soc Sci Med* 1990; 31: 1347–63.

69 Sculpher M, Drummond M, O'Brien B. Effectiveness, efficiency and NICE. *BMJ* 2001; 322: 943–44.

70 Maynard A, Bloor K, Freemantle N. Challenges for the National Institute for Clinical Excellence. *BMJ* 2004; 329: 227–29.

71 Gafni A, Birch S. NICE methodological guidelines and decision making in the National Health Service in England and Wales. *Pharmacoeconomics* 2003; 21: 149–57.

CHAPTER 6

The role of health economics in decision-making

The aim of this chapter is to discuss the use of health economic techniques as part of the decision-making process in health care services. It includes a discussion of how health economic evaluations are utilised but also adopts a broader perspective and encompasses other approaches and techniques. The first section of the chapter assesses the relationship between health economics and evidence-based health care. Subsequent sections examine the extent to which economic evaluations are utilised and how budget impact analysis, programme budgeting and marginal analysis can prove to be very useful techniques for decision-makers and in establishing priorities in health care.

Health economics and evidence-based health care

As was highlighted in Chapter 1, the nature of the health care dilemma, with ever-increasing demands placed on health care services against constraints on the resources available to meet them, continues to be a major headache for those at all levels of policymaking, decision-making, commissioning services and the provision and delivery of health care services. The development of policies and strategies based on what has been shown to be clinically effective has been advocated for some time, while terms such as evidence-based health care and clinical effectiveness are now common usage in health care circles. The need to ensure that limited resources are channelled into effective interventions has provided additional impetus to the drive towards evidence-based practice, coupled by claims that the way to reduce cost pressures in health care is to focus on proven quality.[1]

The relationship between health economics and evidence-based medicine is one that has aroused interest among health economists[2-4] and leading proponents of evidence-based health care.[5] The establishment of the Cochrane Centre in 1992, and subsequently the Cochrane Collaboration in 1993, can be traced back to the publication of the Rock Carling Fellowship Lecture by Archie Cochrane, entitled 'Effectiveness and efficiency: random reflections on health services'.[6] To some extent, it could be argued that the evidence-based medicine and evidence-based health care agendas have focused on the first of these 'Es' – effectiveness, with efficiency not featuring as prominently and equity considerations being excluded.[2] However, Cochrane himself recognised the importance of cost,[6] while others have also stressed the significance of cost and resource issues within an evidence-based health care context.[5,7,8] For example, in seeking to minimise the extent of the conflict between a doctor's responsibilities to the individual patient and responsibilities to society, there are six potential strategies, all of which require 'more and better evidence'.[5] They are:

(1) Eliminate useless or harmful clinical manoeuvres.
(2) Expand effective, cost-saving clinical manoeuvres.
(3) Use equally effective but less expensive alternative clinical manoeuvres.
(4) Determine and apply the cost-utility properties of clinical manoeuvres.
(5) Inform the public.
(6) Be explicit about the presence and nature of conflicts.

It has also been suggested that equality – albeit a narrow perspective – was also one of the guiding concepts (along with effectiveness and efficiency) that influenced Cochrane.[9] In fact, Alan Williams proposed that, in the attempts to move forward with the effectiveness and efficiency agendas, equality and equity should be given a 'greater, but equally searching, share of the limelight'.[9]

Recently, the use of economics alongside Cochrane-type reviews has been illustrated as being potentially useful for decision-makers, without necessarily having to go the 'whole hog' in terms of full cost-per-QALY estimation.[4,10] This seems an eminently sensible approach, and while there may be differences in approaches, methodologies and goals there is scope for 'more fusion than fission'.[11]

What has been advocated is the use of a decision matrix, as shown in Figure 6.1, where outcome measures of different levels of sophistication are introduced,[4,10] and where the importance of trade-offs are recognised and decision-makers are forced to earn their crust without getting too involved with the technical details associated with modelling approaches and which are a potential turn-off for decision-makers.

Despite the emphasis on evidence relating to both effectiveness and cost-effectiveness in policy documentation, it will only bear fruit in practice if relevant research findings and valid guideline recommendations become part of normal practice, and organisational environments are adjusted to facilitate such approaches. The multifaceted complexities of organisational cultures and politics are compounded by the variability in personalities, of which they are composed, and which all combine to produce a spectrum of outcomes that may range from explosive failures to highly successful programmes and policies. More work needs to be undertaken to assess the effectiveness of intraorganisational, interorganisational, interprofessional, collaborative and partnership approaches to the organisation and delivery of services,[12,13] in order to accompany the wealth of research evidence relating to effectiveness and efficiency.

		Declining effectiveness			
		1	2	3	4
	A	y	y	j	n
	B	y	y/n	n	n
	C	j	n	n	n
	D	n	n	n	n

y = yes adopt
n = no reject
y/n = indifferent
j = judgement needed

Effectiveness
Compared with control the intervention has:
1 evidence of greater effectiveness
2 evidence of no difference in effectiveness
3 evidence of less effectiveness
4 not enough evidence of effectiveness

Cost
Compared with control the intervention has:
A evidence of cost savings
B evidence of no difference in costs
C evidence of greater costs
D not enough evidence on costs

Figure 6.1 Integration of effectiveness and resource utilisation evidence. (*Source*: Based on Donaldson *et al.*[10])

There are also other costs associated with the application of evidence that need to be mentioned. The jungle of journals delivered to every practitioner in the course of a week and the volume of material available on the Internet add to the already severe pressures on them to read, appraise and determine their relevance to their particular situations. This obviously presupposes that the desire to adopt and utilise evidence-based information is present. However, it has been demonstrated that 'the naive assumption that when research information is made available it is somehow accessed by practitioners, appraised and then applied in practice is now largely discredited'.[14] Indeed, it has been argued that much research appears to have very little or no impact on practice, and to think about the use of research evidence without considering the organisational context is to miss a good part of the story.[15] Decision-makers need to remove impediments to new ways of working and more often to supply supportive structures, which incorporate and sustain new initiatives and activities if the benefits resulting from evidence-based health care and health economics are to accrue.[15] A further issue arises from the translation of evidence from research into everyday health care practice. The problems associated with generalisability of economic evaluations were discussed in Chapter 5, but caution needs to be exercised in applying the findings from clinical trials, with economic evaluations bolted on, and carried out in controlled conditions, over a limited timescale to everyday situations with 'normal' patients. It has been shown that in applied trial-based cost-effectiveness studies, few provide sufficient evidence for decision-makers to establish the relevance or to adjust the results of the study to their location of interest.[16] Furthermore, it has been argued that the complexities and potential conflicts which exist within organisations at any one point in time make it compulsory to know not only what works but also why and in what circumstances it works or does not work.[17] The ratio of costs and benefits in applying evidence is a crucial factor. If the costs of changing behaviour are greater than the benefits resulting from change, it may be preferable to retain the status quo. Because of the workings of health care systems, new, important and cost-effective treatments sometimes do not become routine care, while well-marketed products of equivocal value may achieve widespread adoption, especially if recommended by a funding agency.[18] The question has been asked whether managers should attempt to influence clinical behaviour and adjust for these inefficient practices, but the conclusion was reached that trying to improve the uptake of underused cost-effective care or reduce the overuse of new and expensive treatments may not always make economic sense in terms of the cost-benefit ratio.[19]

The use of health economic evaluations

Chapter 5 highlighted the nature and ideal structure of economic evaluations. As was discussed, while the use of such evaluations is increasing there remains considerable scepticism as to their relevance and role in the assessment and evaluation of health care technologies and programmes. Studies have attempted to assess the extent to which economic evaluations in health care are used by decision-makers and have concluded that, while the importance of information relating to costs and cost-effectiveness is highly important, issues relating to the accessibility, generalisability, validity and quality of health economic studies represent major obstacles to increasing their usage and contribution to the decision-making process.[20–24] It has been suggested that a potential way forward is to increase awareness and improve the quality of health economic evaluation databases,[21] and a project funded by the European Commission has been established with this in mind.[25] However, general practitioners have suggested, albeit in a small-scale study of 27 GPs in the West of Scotland, that precise, locally generated information on cost-effectiveness would be helpful which would not necessarily be served by national or international databases.[20] However, the difficulties and resources needed to produce such information may well be prohibitive, although the efforts to secure specific data for their populations have been strongly advocated by AWMSG and SMC in recent years.

A further problem arises as a result of the quality of many economic evaluations undertaken in health care. For example, in 326 submissions made by the pharmaceutical industry for funding in Australia, 67% had significant problems,[26] while less than one-third of studies considered in a systematic review of health economic evaluations in gastroenterology met the criteria established for being of high quality.[27]

The difficulties involved in utilising evidence relating to the cost-effectiveness of interventions can be seen in the area of multiple sclerosis, where there has been considerable activity, debate and discussion over a number of years as to the extent to which disease-modifying agents could be regarded as being cost-effective.[28] For example, in 1997, the question was asked whether in the case of interferon-β in multiple sclerosis costs could be controlled.[29] This led to correspondence between the manufacturing company and the authors of the article,[30,31] which in some senses set the tone for what was to follow in the literature and as government agencies deliberated whether to 'fund' the provision of these therapies.

In the UK, for example, the report written for the Department of Health Health Technology Assessment Programme[32] set the scene for the appraisal undertaken by NICE.[33] This involved a lengthy and tortuous process of appraisal, appeal and reappraisal of available and emerging evidence, the outcome of which is the risk-sharing scheme proposed by the UK Department of Health, currently being trialled. Much of the debate centred on the modelling approaches employed. The wide range of estimates reflects the difficulties inherent in translating the results from clinical trials into models that aim to assess the cost-effectiveness of interventions in chronic disease management, while the lack of homogeneity in the design of the studies also contributes to the wide variation in the estimates of cost-effectiveness and the difficulty of arriving at a consensus. Short-term analyses avoid the problems of attempting to extrapolate from clinical data, but fail to do justice to the duration of the illness and its progression over time, while longer-term studies may capture the longer-term effects, but do so with only limited evidence to substantiate the extrapolations from relatively short-term data and the assumptions underlying the construction of the models. While recent studies have benefited from more relevant and up-to-date data relating to disease progression,[34–38] uncertainty in the actual scale of benefit gained from the interventions in terms of delayed progression of disability continues to affect attempts at estimating cost-effectiveness.[34]

In summary, the complexity of the disease and its progression, inconclusive evidence on the effectiveness of the agents and their impact on progression, the methodological issues in assessing the cost-effectiveness of interventions in multiple sclerosis and in chronic diseases in general, have all contributed to making the issue one that has provided more than its fair share of debate and discussion in the literature. What is clearly evident is that there is a need for further research to establish 'robust and stable outcome measures', to 'obtain real data on the progress of people once they have stopped treatment'[34] 'to identify those who will benefit most from disease-modifying treatments'.[39]

Requirements for health economic evaluations

The growth in the number of health economic evaluations has led to the development of guidelines for the conduct, design and methodology of such studies. A number of countries (e.g. Australia, Canada, Finland, New Zealand, Norway) have made submission of economic evaluations an official requirement for placement of medication on their national formulary while others (e.g. Denmark, France) have encouraged such submissions. In the UK, NICE expects companies to submit a dossier of evidence of clinical effectiveness and cost-effectiveness relating to their product when an assessment of that particular technology is being undertaken. An example is shown in Box 6.1.[40]

Box 6.1 Requirements for health economics evaluations

Study design
1. The research question is stated
2. The economic importance of the research question is stated
3. The viewpoint(s) of the analysis are clearly stated and justified
4. The rationale for choosing the alternative programmes or interventions compared is stated
5. The alternatives being compared are clearly described
6. The form of economic evaluation used is stated
7. The choice of form of economic evaluation is justified in relation to the questions addressed

Data collection
8. The source(s) of effectiveness estimates used are stated
9. Details of the design and results of effectiveness study are given (if based on a single study)
10. Details of the method of synthesis or meta-analysis of estimates are given (if based on an overview of a number of effectiveness studies)
11. The primary outcome measure(s) for the economic evaluation are clearly stated
12. Methods to value health states and other benefits are stated
13. Details of the subjects from whom valuations were obtained are given
14. Productivity changes (if included) are reported separately
15. The relevance of productivity changes to the study question is discussed
16. Quantities of resources are reported separately from their unit costs

Continued

Box 6.1 Requirements for health economics evaluations —*Continued*

17. Methods for the estimation of quantities and unit costs are described
18. Currency and price data are recorded
19. Details of currency of price adjustments for inflation or currency conversion are given
20. Details of any model used are given
21. The choice of model used and the key parameters on which it is based are justified

Analysis and interpretation of results

22. Time horizon of costs and benefits is stated
23. The discount rate(s) is stated
24. The choice of rate(s) is justified
25. An explanation is given if costs or benefits are not discounted
26. Details of statistical tests and confidence intervals are given for stochastic data
27. The approach to sensitivity analysis is given
28. The choice of variables for sensitivity analysis is justified
29. The ranges over which the variables are varies are stated
30. Relevant alternatives are compared
31. Incremental analysis is reported
32. Major outcomes are presented in a disaggregated as well as aggregated form
33. The answer to the study question is given
34. Conclusions follow from the data reported
35. Conclusions are accompained by the appropriate caveats

Source: Derived from Durummond and Jefferson.[40]

The use of economic evaluation in decision-making

The use of health economic evaluations has grown enormously in recent years and could be regarded as constituting an industry in its own right with the advent of pharmacoeconomics. Pharmaceutical interventions are assessed in relation to their cost-effectiveness relative to current therapies or other alternative treatments, and then form the basis for submissions to reimbursement bodies for approval and funding. As a result the pharmaceutical industry has established specific departments, usually under the banner of Outcomes Research, which undertake economic evaluations and provide other health economics advice, for example in relation to pricing. There has also been a burgeoning in the number of consultancy firms offering advice and support to the pharmaceutical industry on issues relating to health economics. The discipline has certainly made vast strides and grown exponentially since the publication of the seminal work by Alan Williams 'The

Economics of Coronary Artery Bypass Grafting'.[41] However, major problems still remain.

NICE, AWMSG, SMC, and economic evaluations

Reference has been made throughout the book to NICE. It was set up as a Special Health Authority for England and Wales on 1 April 1999 to provide patients, health professionals and the public with authoritative, robust and reliable guidance on current 'best practice'. The role of NICE has been, to some degree, controversial. Its appraisal of new technologies and attempts to provide guidance on what constitutes 'best practice' have not been without its detractors.[18,42–45] Its processes involve assessing the clinical evidence relating to medications and therapies, as well as the evidence relating to the cost-effectiveness of such interventions, to produce guidance for decision-makers within the NHS as to whether such treatments should be made widely available. For example, the key recommendations of the NICE review on PPIs for dyspepsia are highlighted in Box 6.2.

Box 6.2 Guidance on the Use of Proton Pump Inhibitors in the Treatment of Dyspepsia

Category of dyspepsia	Recommendations
Peptic ulcer	Patients with documented duodenal or gastric ulcers should be tested for *Helicobacter Pylori* (HP) and, if positive, should have received eradication therapy – usually a PPI and two antibiotics in high dose for 7 days. If they remain symptomatic after eradication, or are HP-negative, they should receive a healing dose of PPI, and once healing has been achieved, treatment should be stepped down to the lowest effective dose or stopped.
NSAID-induced ulcers	Patients with documented NSAID-induced ulcers should receive a healing dose of a PPI, followed by a step-down to a maintenance dose, which may be given long term.
Gastro-oesophageal reflux disease (GORD)	Patients with severe GORD should be treated with a healing dose of PPI to achieve symptom control followed by a step-down to a maintenance dose. Patients with oesophageal strictures should not be stepped down and should be maintained on healing doses to reduce risk of restricturing.

Continued

Box 6.2 Guidance on the Use of Proton Pump Inhibitors in the Treatment of Dyspepsia—*Continued*

	Patients with mild GORD can be managed on less expensive therapies, using acid suppressants or antacids to control symptoms.
Non-ulcer dyspepsia	Patients with non-ulcer dyspepsia should be treated with a step-up or step-down at the lowest dosage to control symptoms, but that they should not be treated with long-term PPIs unless their use is confirmed by endoscopy.

Source: NICE.[46]

It should be noted that the guidance issued by NICE on PPIs has now been updated and subsumed within its Clinical Guidelines on Dyspepsia.[47] There has been much discussion about the role of NICE and how it reaches its conclusions, and uncertainty about the impact of guidance on the NHS and about who monitors compliance.[43] Authorities are required to provide appropriate funding for treatments recommended by NICE within 3 months of the announcement, which may well result in other services being denied funding[48] and the geographical inequities, which NICE was intended to reduce and remove, being switched to other services. In addition, there have been claims that NICE is inherently inflationary[18] and, as highlighted in Chapter 5, recent controversy has centred on whether NICE has a threshold cost-per-QALY criterion.[49,50]

The remit of the Scottish Medicines Consortium (SMC) is shown in Box 6.3 and that of the All Wales Medicines Strategy Group (AWMSG) in Box 6.4.

The modus operandi of AWMSG and SMC is different from that of NICE. The SMC requires all newly licensed products, new formulations of existing medications and major new indications for current products to be submitted for assessment. In Wales, one of the roles of AWMSG is to review all new drugs, indications and formulations and appraise new high-cost therapeutic developments. AWMSG considers new medicines that are likely to cost the NHS in Wales more than £2000 per patient per year, or more than £2000 per patient per year when associated indirect costs are taken into account. Drugs that are low in cost but high in volume are also within AWMSG's remit for assessment. However, AWMSG does not in any way duplicate or conflict with the work of NICE, which has ultimate responsibility for guiding medical practice in England and Wales. Advice issued by NICE would supercede any guidance issues by AWMSG. The role of AWMSG is to provide interim guidance for drugs that have yet to be appraised by NICE, or for drugs that may have been appraised, but for which publication is some time away.

Box 6.3 Remit of the Scottish Medicines Consortium

The remit of the Scottish Medicines Consortium (SMC) is to provide advice to NHS Boards and their Area Drug and Therapeutics Committees (ADTCs) across Scotland about the status of all newly licensed medicines, all new formulations of existing medicines and any major new indications for established products. The review of medicines containing devices will be confined to those licensed as medicines by the MHRA/EMEA. This remit covers all new products licensed from January 2002. This advice will be made available as soon as practical after the launch of the product involved. SMC has formed a sub-working group named the New Drugs Committee (NDC) which will advise and make recommendations on the issues surrounding newly licensed products to the SMC.

The SMC Process requires pharmaceutical companies to complete a New Product Submission form. The aim is to make a recommendation soon after the launch of a product. The timescales involved require the submission to be made ahead of product launch.

Source: *http://www.scottishmedicines.org.uk* (accessed 12 January 2005)

NICE has a series of programmes, referred to as waves, within which a series of appraisals will be undertaken. The technologies themselves are formally referred to NICE by the Secretary of State for Health and the Welsh Assembly Government, and the process from referral to final appeal takes a minimum of 54 weeks. The NICE process is much more involved and detailed than its Scottish and Welsh counterparts, and in terms of its effectiveness the jury is still very much out.[44,45,50,51] For example, in its guidance on PPIs for dyspepsia it concluded that 'a reduction in PPI usage of up to 15% could be produced if doctors were to review indications, reduce dosages to appropriate levels and use the least expensive appropriate PPI. . . . The resultant savings would be between £40 [million] and £50 million per year'.[46] However, in the Assessment Report that underpinned their guidance on Cox II inhibitors[52] the following statement is made in relation to the costs associated with adverse events relating to NSAIDs:

> Moore *et al.* estimate that the annual burden of NSAID-related GI side effects to the NHS is £251m.–367m. This includes the direct hospital costs (£36m. p.a.) and prophylactic co-prescriptions of PCA (£130m.–331m. p.a.).[53]

The prescribing of gastroprotective agents costs the NHS between 3 and 7 times as much as potential savings from using least expensive PPIs as recommended by NICE and lends weight to some of the claims that focusing solely on the cost-effectiveness of specific interventions fails to take into account some of the broader issues surrounding the allocation of resources.

Box 6.4 Remit of the All Wales Medicines Strategy Group

The All Wales Medicines Strategy Group (AWMSG) will provide advice to the Minister for Health and Social Services in an effective, efficient and transparent manner on strategic medicines management and prescribing. The AWMSG, acting in a strategic and advisory capacity, will be seen as the conduit through which consensus can be reached on medicines management issues, especially those affecting both primary and secondary care.

The Group's main functions will be to:

- Advise the Assembly of future developments in health care to assist in its strategic planning.
- Develop timely, independent and authoritative advice on new drugs and on the cost implications of making these drugs routinely available on the NHS.
- Advise the Assembly on the development of a prescribing strategy for Wales.
- Advise the Assembly on the implementation of a range of strategic Prescribing Task and Finish Group recommendations.

The AWMSG Process requires pharmaceutical companies to complete a Therapeutic Development Appraisal Form. The aim is to make a recommendation soon after the launch of a product. The timescales involved require the submission to be made ahead of product launch.

Source: *http://www.wales.nhs.uk/sites/home.cfm?OrgID=371* (accessed 12 January 2005)

On the other hand, the attitude of the Audit Commission, which offered the following view, is more encouraging:

> In recent years, these cost pressures have been driven by the introduction of new medicines. . . . These cost pressures are cause for concern for many Trust boards, but they need to be viewed as part of the overall package of patient care. For some conditions, medicines expenditure should be rising because it would be a cost-effective way of increasing the health gain for the population. For example, expenditure on proton pump inhibitors and H2 antagonists should be rising because their use improves the quality of patients' lives and saves money by preventing invasive surgery.[54]

The establishment and development of agencies such as AWMSG, NICE and SMC has cemented the role of health economic evaluations in relation to decision-making in health care. However, economic evaluations can be used for rather perverse reasons as well. The tobacco giant, Philip Morris, undertook a cost-benefit analysis of smoking for the Treasury of the Czech Republic in 1999. It compared the costs of increased medical care for smokers and time lost through tobacco-related health problems against the income gained from taxes on tobacco and the money saved to pension funds and housing costs due to premature mortality resulting from smoking, and concluded that smoking resulted in a net gain of $224 million![55]

The use of health economics and decision-making

Another requirement of submissions made to the relevant assessment agency is that of an estimation of the resource requirements that the intervention would involve. For example, AWMSG and SMC ask manufacturers to provide responses to the questions posed in Box 6.5.

The problems associated with budgets and their management have been discussed in Chapter 3, while the issues associated with determining the impact of services and interventions on budgets were briefly considered in Chapter 2. Health economic evaluations do not take into consideration situations that arise when expenditure in one budget area brings about savings in another. Savings resulting from interventions in one budget area cannot be passed on to the budget area that incurred the expenditure. For example, the

---

Box 6.5 Estimation of Resource Requirements (based on AWMSG and SMC forms)

(a) Please give an estimate of the total number of patients who have the condition relating to the indication under consideration (current prevalence), and an indication of the source of estimated numbers.

(b) Please give an estimate of the number of newly diagnosed patients each year over the first 5 years after introduction (yearly incidence), and an indication of the source of estimated numbers.

(c) If appropriate, please give an estimate of the net number of patients in each of the first 5 years after introduction. (net number = prevalent cases + incident cases – patients who recover or die).

(d) Give an estimate of the number of people currently treated for this condition.

(e) Give an estimate of the number of people likely to be prescribed this treatment, with the basis for calculation.

(f) For the product under consideration in this submission, and for the principal alternative treatments, give the direct cost associated with treatment over a defined time period.

(g) For the product under consideration in this submission, identify any direct savings over a defined time period.

(h) Provide a summary of the net resource implications in each of the first 5 years following introduction. This should take account of acquisition costs associated with the new treatment and with other therapy whose uptake may be influenced by its availability.

use of a new therapy in patients being treated in primary care and that would result in fewer emergency hospitalisations, or the need for outpatient follow-up attendances in secondary care, would be financed out of primary care drug budgets. In addition, the benefits of health care provision and improvements in the health of individuals extend way beyond the realms of health care budgets, and savings that accrue to employers, for example, are not passed on to the health service. Questions relating to what the purpose and role of health services are spring to mind at this juncture, with cynics asking whether health services exist to manage financial budgets or to manage patients and their health problems or, in broader terms, the health of the population.

However, it is an increasingly regular feature of the requirements placed on those organisations seeking approval for their new therapies or services from assessment agencies or reimbursement bodies. Some useful qualities that should be present in a budget-impact analysis have been suggested[56] and highlighted in Box 6.6.

The limitations of health economic evaluations, together with the time and resources involved in their production, mean that while they can provide useful information relating to specific interventions or programmes, they are

---

Box 6.6 Characteristics of Budget-Impact Analysis

Transparency – to ensure that all assumptions and relationships between inputs and outcomes are explicit;

Clarity of perspective – usually that of the 'overall' purchaser, but on some occasions it may be possible to disaggregate the impact on total budgets to specific purchasers;

Reliability of data – sources should be clearly stated along with comments relating to their relevance and assumptions made;

Relationship between intermediate and final end points – the ability of clinical trials to predict long-term outcomes is limited and, as with assessing cost-effectiveness, there is need to rely on modelling for such purposes;

Rates of adoption of new therapies – it is often difficult to predict the extent to which new therapies will replace existing ones, while it is also problematic to predict the impact of induced demand resulting from the increased awareness among clinicians and the public. For example, the government's concern over Viagra and other so-called 'lifestyle drugs' and their uptake led to claims that they may even threaten the financial sustainability of current health systems[57];

Impact of intervention by population subgroups or indications – cost-effectiveness studies can be particularly useful here by identifying groups that stand to benefit most from the introduction of new therapies, while at the same time considering the resource implications of treating the groups;

Continued

Box 6.6 Characteristics of Budget-Impact Analysis—*Continued*

Reporting of results – the results should be made available in both natural and monetary units so that the full resource impact can be contemplated, e.g. when new therapies may result in additional GP consultations or district nurse visits;

Re-deploying resources – reductions in bed-days or nursing time are extremely difficult to translate into actual cost reductions, since, in the short-term, the resources are used elsewhere. In the longer-term there may be scope for the realisation of resources over time and budget impact models should provide some indication of these;

Time horizon – from the perspective of budget holders a 1-year impact is desirable along with longer-term assessments. As seen in Box 6.4, AWMSG and SMC request the impact for the first 5 years following introduction;

Dealing with uncertainty – there is likely to be considerable uncertainty within budget-impact models and therefore there should be a section where a sensitivity analysis is provided;

Access to the model – whenever possible decision-makers should be allowed access to the models to test assumptions and to insert local data etc., while recognising any commercial sensitivity that may exist.

---

of less use in the context of decision-making, especially in relation to making choices as to where additional resources should be placed, or which areas should bear the brunt of any cutbacks, within health care organisations.

A technique that has been widely used in such situations is that of programme budgeting and marginal analysis (PBMA). Programme budgeting focuses on the outputs and outcomes of services in relation to the inputs used to generate such outputs and outcomes. The critical difference between programme budgeting and other types of budgeting rests in the emphasis given to the relationship between inputs and outputs/outcomes rather than concentrating on the inputs required. Programme budgeting, on its own, would not be a suitable technique for determining priorities. However, the incorporation of marginal analysis alongside programme budgeting does provide a 'framework to explore ways of improving the technical efficiency of programmes by examining the cost-effectiveness of the mix of inputs'[58], and 'by considering opportunity costs at the margin, decision-makers can improve service delivery options within the constraint of limited resources', while at the same time recognising and taking into account the complexities and different agendas impacting on health care decision-making.[59]

The concept of the 'margin' was considered in Chapter 3 and is extremely important in economics. It focuses on the additional unit of a service and the cost of producing that particular unit and the benefits generated by that unit. It is thus possible to determine the extent of resources to be allocated to a variety of different programmes and ensure that the benefits generated cannot be exceeded. This is when the marginal benefit/marginal cost ratio is the same across all programmes. If this ratio is 4:1 in Programme A and 2:1 in Programme B, a reallocation of resources from Programme B to Programme A would result in a net increase in benefits generated by both programmes. However, if both programmes had a ratio of 3:1, a reallocation of resources from one programme to the other would mean a net decrease in benefits. Maximum benefit will be achieved when the marginal benefit/marginal cost ratio is the same across all programmes or subprogrammes.

There are a number of examples where PBMA has been employed.[60–66] The basic approach of PBMA has been well documented and interested readers are invited to read the tool kit provided by Mitton and Donaldson.[59] There are subtle differences in the approaches offered by different authors, but in summary, PBMA can be depicted in a series of stages.

Stage 1: to determine the aim and scope of the priority-setting programme, which basically provides the terms of reference for the exercise and identifies a set of meaningful programmes with which to work – for example, age groups, disease groups or clinical directorate groups. There are no hard and fast rules as to what actually constitutes a programme other than it must be output- or outcome-orientated and preferably disaggregated into subprogrammes.

Stage 2: to map current activity levels and expenditure in relation to the identified programmes and ensure that the total budget is reflected, so as to avoid omissions and items being double counted. This in essence provides the baseline from where the process actually commences and becomes extremely important later in the process when the implications of switching resources are considered.

Stage 3: to set up an advisory panel and use it to determine the relevant decision-making criteria, against which the implications of resource reallocations can be assessed. Despite the limitations of information relating to benefits, this stage helps define a programme and subprogrammes, and enables a view to be taken of the expenditures incurred and benefits yielded before any consideration is given to the implications of moving resources.

Stage 4: to consider the options as to which programmes and subprogrammes should expand, which programmes and subprogrammes could achieve similar levels of activity for a smaller resource envelope, and which programmes and subprogrammes could release resources by reducing levels of activity or stopping them altogether.

Stage 5: where the impact of proposed changes takes place, and where marginal analysis has a role to play. The advisory panel would make recommendations as to how the growth areas are to be financed, out of new additional resources, or from resources released by achieving similar levels of activity for fewer resources, or by curtailing or stopping some programmes and subprogrammes.

> The implications of resource switching from one programme or subprogramme to another can be gauged against the criteria identified under Stage 2 and the recommendations made accordingly.

The beauty of such an approach lies in its transparency, and in a public sector service like the NHS, it is unlikely that there will be complete unanimity of views, but decisions will nevertheless have to be made. PBMA is a good way to lay the whole process out to public scrutiny. It is important, however, that the changes are well managed and subjected to ongoing monitoring and evaluation.

It is not advocated, however, that PBMA is problem-free and a number of problems have been highlighted:

- the time and information requirements may well prove to be a major constraint in undertaking PBMA;
- the need to have a multidisciplinary approach to PBMA compounds the time problem and the results of the exercise may be highly dependent upon the composition of the expert group[58];
- the asymmetry of information between providers and purchasers may result in possible contention in determining when to involve providers in the PBMA process, which can also result in excessive reliance on the literature on the part of purchasers[67];
- the lack of relevant local evidence with regard to some of the criteria, and good quality data on outcomes, may force the use of intermediate outputs, the maximisation of which may have detrimental effects elsewhere, for example, seeking to maximise consultant episodes may result in patients being discharged too early[68];
- PBMA may produce findings that are too broad to be of any practical value. The role of the advisory group in deciding which areas should be considered in the analysis may lead 'to an inconsistency in applying the rigour of economic evaluations to options that have been selected in a way that is essentially arbitrary' and the results of economic evaluations may be biased 'if the range of options selected for evaluation excludes viable alternatives'.[58] A flow diagram approach has been advocated that maps potential patient flows through the health care system and identifies decision points where alternative service options are (or may be) available. The role of the group is thus concentrated on developing the flow diagram and highlighting sources of data rather than indicating the areas they wish to consider in the analysis. This, they suggest, excludes the use of PBMA as a bargaining exercise and enhances its capability as a means of evaluating the resource and outcome consequences of all relevant options.[58]

However, despite its limitations, a number of PBMA studies have been undertaken with varying degrees of success, which lends weight to the view that the criticisms should be kept in perspective and considered as a means of securing improvements in the process. It has been argued that 'application of the marginal-analysis framework appears to offer a clear improvement in the way priorities are set'[63] and the recent directory of

PBMA exercises, studies and publications bears testimony to the improvements that have been made and the usefulness of the approach.[59]

Health policy issues are high on political agendas. Technological advancements, developments in medical science and increasing expectations of communities as to what is available from health care providers continue to focus attention on the health care dilemma. Choices will always have to be made regarding the level of resources allocated to health care and, within health care, regarding which areas should receive a greater share and which areas less. In making such choices an explicit set of priorities needs to be established and attitudes changed. The evidence base for the effectiveness of interventions and management strategies is continuously being developed. The recognition of the need to generate evidence relating to resource utilisation and the most beneficial utilisation of available resources is encouraging. However, the existence of ineffectiveness and inefficiencies in service provision has to be addressed. The development of evidence-based practice, a recognition that resources are finite and that choices have to be made, and an awareness of the need for fairness in resource allocation and service provision are major steps along the road to answering the question of how much additional resources should be put into health care in general. The technical problems surrounding economic approaches to priority setting should not be allowed to detract from the fact that they provide a rational framework within which other issues, such as considerations of equity and public and professional opinion, can be embraced and priorities established. However crude the techniques and tools of health economics, attempts to set priorities within the context of a transparent and relatively rational framework 'should be welcomed as a challenge to the covert, imprecise and inconsistent practice of prioritisation which exists in all health care systems today'.[69]

References

1 Marwick C. Proponents gather together to discuss practicing evidence-based medicine. *JAMA* 1997; 278: 531–32.
2 Maynard A. Evidence-based medicine: cost effectiveness and equity are ignored. *BMJ* 1996; 313: 170.
3 Birch S. Making the problem fit the solution: evidence-based economics decision making and 'Dolly' economics, in Donaldson C, Mugford M, Vale L (eds). *Evidence-based health economics: from effectiveness to efficiency in systematic review.* London: BMJ Books, 2002.
4 Vale L, Donaldson C, Daly C *et al.* Evidence-based medicine and health economics: a case study of end stage renal disease. *Health Econ* 2000; 9: 337–51.
5 Sackett DL. *The doctor's (ethical and economic) dilemma.* London: Office of Health Economics, 1996.
6 Cochrane AL. *Effectiveness and efficiency: random reflections on health services.* London: Nuffield Provincial Hospitals Trust, 1972.
7 Muir Gray JA. *Evidence-based healthcare.* Edinburgh: Churchill Livingstone, 1997.

8 Moore A. Waste in the NHS: the problem, its size and how we can tackle it. *Bandolier Extra* 2002. *http://www.jr2.ox.ac.uk/bandolier/Extraforbando/Waste.pdf* (accessed 16 Ocotber 2004)

9 Williams A. Beyond effectiveness and efficiency...lies equality! in Maynard A, Chalmers I (eds). *Non-random reflections of health services research: on the 25th anniversary of Archie Cochrane's 'Effectiveness and Efficiency'.* London: BMJ Books, 1997.

10 Donaldson C, Mugford M, Vale L (eds). *Evidence-based health economics: from effectiveness to systematic review.* London: BMJ Books, 2002.

11 Drummond M. Evidence-based medicine meets economic evaluation: an agenda for research, in Donaldson C, Mugford M, Vale L (eds). *Evidence-based health economics: from effectiveness to systematic review.* London: BMJ Books, 2002.

12 El Ansari W, Phillips CJ, Hammick M. Collaboration and partnerships: developing the evidence base. *Health Soc Care Commun* 2001; 9: 215–27.

13 El Ansari W, Phillips CJ. Interprofessional collaboration: a stakeholder approach to evaluation of voluntary participation in community partnerships. *J Interprofession Care* 2001; 15: 351–68.

14 NHS Centre for Reviews and Disssemination. *Getting research into practice.* Effective Health Care Bulletin 5: 1. London: Royal Society of Medicine Press, 1999.

15 Weiss CH. Have we learned anything new about the use of evaluation? *Am J Eval* 1998; 19: 21–33.

16 Sculpher MJ, Pang FS, Manca A *et al.* Generalisability in economic evaluation studies in healthcare: a review and case studies. *Health Technol Assess* 2004; 8: 1–206.

17 Pawson R, Tilley N. *Realistic evaluation.* London: Sage, 1997.

18 Maynard A, Bloor K, Freemantle N. Challenges for the National Institute for Clinical Excellence. *BMJ* 2004; 329: 227–29.

19 Mason J, Freemantle N, Nazareth I *et al.* When is it cost-effective to change the behavior of health professionals? *JAMA* 2001; 286: 2988–92.

20 Wu O, Knill-Jones R, Wilson P *et al.* The impact of economic information on medical decision making in primary care. *J Eval Clin Pract* 2004; 10: 407–11.

21 Hoffman C, Graf von der Schulenburg JM. The influence of economic evaluation studies on decision making: a European survey. *Health Policy* 2000; 52: 179–92.

22 Drummond MF, Cooke J, Walley T. Economic evaluation under managed competition: evidence from the UK. *Soc Sci Med* 1997; 45: 583–95.

23 Duthie T, Trueman P, Chancellor J *et al.* Research into the use of health economics in decision making in the United Kingdom – Phase II: is health economics 'for good or evil'? *Health Policy* 1999; 46: 143–57.

24 Hoffman C, Stoykova BA, Nixon J *et al.* Do health-care decision makers find health economic evaluations useful? The findings of focus group research in UK health authorities. *Value Health* 2002; 592: 71–79.

25 Drummond MF. Making economic evaluations more accessible to health care decision-makers. *Eur J Health Econ* 2003; 4: 246–47.

26 Hill S, Mitchell AS, Henry DA. Problems with the interpretation of pharmacoeconomic analysis: a review of submissions to the Australian Pharmaceutical Benefits Scheme. *JAMA* 2000; 283: 2116–21.

27 Speigel BMR, Targownik LE, Kanwal F *et al.* The quality of published health economic analyses in digestive diseases: a systematic review and quantitative appraisal. *Gastroenterology* 2004; 127: 403–11.

28 Phillips CJ. The cost-effectiveness of disease-modifying agents in the treatment of multiple sclerosis. *CNS Drugs* 2004; 18: 561–74.

29 Tolley KH, Whynes DK. Interferon-β in multiple sclerosis: can we control its costs? *Pharmacoeconomics* 1997; 11: 210–15.

30 Madgwick T. Response to Tolley KH, Whynes DK. *Pharmacoeconomics* 1997; 12: 499–500.

31 Tolley KH, Whynes DK. Reply to Madgwick T. *Pharmacoeconomics* 1997; 12: 500–501.

32 Parkin D, McNamee P, Jacoby A *et al.* A cost-utility analysis of interferon beta for multiple sclerosis. *Health Tech Assess* 1998; 2.

33 National Institute for Clinical Excellence. Beta interferon and glatiramer acetate for the treatment of multiple sclerosis. *NICE Technology Appraisal Guidance*, No. 32. *http://www.nice.org.uk/pdf/Multiple%20Sclerosis%20Final%20Guidance.pdf* (accessed 22 December 2004)

34 Nuijten MJC, Hutton J. Cost-effectiveness analysis of interferon beta in multiple sclerosis: a Markov process analysis. *Value Health* 2002; 5: 44–54.

35 Chilcott J, McCabe C, Tappenden P *et al.* Modelling the cost effectiveness of interferon beta and glatiramer acetate in the management of multiple sclerosis. *BMJ* 2003; 326: 522.

36 Kobelt G, Jönsson L, Fredrikson S. Cost-utility of interferon ß$_{1b}$ 1-b in the treatment of patients with active relapsing-remiting or secondary progressive multiple sclerosis. *Eur J Health Econ* 2003; 4: 50–59.

37 Phillips CJ, Gilmour L, Gale R *et al.* A cost utility model of beta-interferon in the treatment of relapsing-remitting multiple sclerosis. *J Med Econ* 2001; 4: 35–50.

38 Kobelt G, Jönsson L, Miltenberger C. Cost-utility of interferon beta 1-b in secondary progressive multiple sclerosis, using natural history disease data. *Int J Technol Assess Health Care* 2002; 18: 127–38.

39 Miller DH. Commentary: evaluating disease-modifying treatments in multiple sclerosis. *BMJ* 2003; 326: 522.

40 Drummond MF, Jefferson TO (on behalf of the BMJ Economic Evaluation Working Party). Guidelines for authors and peer reviewers of economic submissions to the BMJ. *BMJ* 1996; 313: 275–83.

41 Williams A. The economics of coronary artery bypass grafting. *BMJ* 1985; 291: 326–29.

42 Smith R. The failings of NICE. *BMJ* 2000; 321: 1363–64.

43 Dent THS, Sadler M. From guidance to practice: why NICE is not enough. *BMJ* 2002; 324: 842–45.

44 Gafni A, Birch S. NICE methodological guidelines and decision making in the National Health Service in England and Wales. *Pharmacoeconomics* 2003; 21: 149–57.

45 Sheldon TA, Cullum N, Dawson D *et al.* What's the evidence that NICE guidance has been implemented? Results from a national evaluation using time series analysis, audit of patients' notes and interviews. *BMJ* 2004; 329: 999. doi:10.1136/bmj.329.7473.999 (accessed 12 January 2005)

46 NICE. Guidance on the use of proton pump inhibitors in the treatment of dyspepsia. *Technology Appraisal Guidance*, No. 7, July 2000. *http://www.nice.org.uk/pdf/proton.pdf* (accessed 12 January 2005)

47 NICE. Dyspepsia: mangagement of dyspepsia in adults in primary care, *Clinical Guideline*, 17 August 2004. *http://www.nice.org.uk/pdf/CG017NICEguideline.pdf* (accessed 12 January 2005)

48 Sculpher M, Drummond M, O'Brien B. Effectiveness, efficiency and NICE. *BMJ* 2001; 322: 943–44.

49 Towse A, Pritchard C. Does NICE have a threshold? An external view, in Towse A, Pritchard C, Devlin N (eds). *Cost-effectiveness thresholds: economic and ethical issues.* London: Office of Health Economics, 2003.

50 Rawlins M, Culyer AJ. National Institute for Clinical Excellence and its value judgements. *BMJ* 2004; 329: 224–27.

51 Williams A. *What could be nicer than NICE?* London: Office of Health Economics, 2004.

52 NICE. Guidance on the use of cyclo-oxygenase (Cox) II selective inhibitors, celecoxib, rofecoxib, meloxicam and etodolac for osteoarthritis and rheumatoid arthritis. *Technology Appraisal Guidance,* No. 27, July 2001. *http://www.nice.org.uk/pdf/coxiifullguidance.pdf* (accessed 12 January 2005)

53 NICE Appraisal Team. The clinical effectiveness and cost effectiveness of celecoxib, rofecoxib, meloxicam and etodolac (Cox-II inhibitors) for rheumatoid arthritis and osteoarthritis, November 2000. *http://www.nice.org.uk/pdf/coxiihtareport.pdf* (accessed 12 January 2005)

54 Audit Commission. *A spoonful of sugar: medicines management in NHS hospitals.* London: Audit Commission, 2001.

55 Mallenson A. *Whiplash and other useful illnesses.* Montreal: McGill-Queen's University Press, 2002.

56 Trueman P, Drummond M, Hutton J. Developing guidance for budget impact analysis. *Pharmacoeconomics* 2001; 19: 609–21.

57 Gilbert D, Walley T, New B. Lifestyle medicines. *BMJ* 2000; 321: 1341–44.

58 Posnett J, Street A. Programme budgeting and marginal analysis: an approach to priority setting in need of refinement. *J Health Serv Res Policy* 1996; 1: 147–53.

59 Mitton G, Donaldson C. *Priority setting tool kit: a guide to the use of economics in healthcare decision making.* London: BMJ Books, 2004.

60 Cohen D. Marginal analysis in practice: an alternative to needs assessment for contracting health care. *BMJ* 1994; 309: 781–84.

61 Craig N, Parkin D, Gerard K. Clearing the fog on the Tyne: programme budgeting in Newcastle and North Tyneside Health Authority. *Health Policy* 1995; 33: 107–26.

62 Twaddle S, Walker A. Programme budgeting and marginal analysis: application within programmes to assist purchasing in Greater Glasgow Health Board. *Health Policy* 1995; 33: 91–106.

63 Cohen D. Messages from mid-Glamorgan: a multi-programme experiment with marginal analysis. *Health Policy* 1995; 33: 147–56.

64 Brambleby P, Fordham R. *What is PBMA?* London: Hayward Medical Communications, 2003. *http://www.jr2.ox.ac.uk/bandolier/painres/download/whatis/pbma.pdf* (accessed 12 January 2005)

65 Brambleby P, Fordham R. *Implementing PBMA?* London: Hayward Medical Communications, 2003. *http://www.jr2.ox.ac.uk/bandolier/painres/download/whatis/pbmaimp.pdf* (accessed 12 January 2005)

66 Mitton C, Donaldson C. Twenty-five years of programme budgeting and marginal analysis in the health sector. *J Health Serv Res Policy* 2001; 6: 239–48.

67 Donaldson C. Economics, public health and health care purchasing: reinventing the wheel? *Health Policy* 1995; 33: 77–90.

68 Coast J. Efficiency: the economic contribution to priority setting, in Coast J, Donovan J, Frankel S (eds). *Priority setting: the health care debate.* London: Wiley and Sons, 1996.

69 Maynard A. Prioritising health care: dreams and reality, in Malek M (ed). *Setting priorities in health care.* London: Wiley and Sons, 1994.

CHAPTER 7
Considering the way forward

The state of the health service provides a constant forum for discussion and debate, with scores of diagnoses made of its problems and solutions offered for its improvement. There is no single solution to the myriad of issues and problems confronting health care decision-makers. Unfortunately, it is not possible to envisage the health service enjoying the same happy ending that resulted in the film of *The Wizard of Oz*, where Dorothy and her friends also encountered many trials, tribulations, problems and challenges on their journey along the Yellow Brick Road in search of the Wizard. At the end of the road was the Emerald City, where their respective needs were met: Scarecrow received brains; the Lion received courage; and the Tin Woodman received a new heart.

The health service will never be in a position to meet everyone's health care needs, let alone people's wants and desires. The politicians, managers and other officials who run the services veer between trying to contain costs and defusing the anger of patients, families and the electorate for the inadequacies in the services that are provided. Media focus on the pressures and problems rather than the successes does little to remedy the situation, while professionals' frustration and anger with what they see as the inadequacies in the system and its effects on patient care are increasingly apparent.

However, the situation is likely to get worse, as half of all health care spending goes on the health care needs of people over 65. Utilisation rates of services in all sectors of the health service are noticeably higher in this age group than in people below the age of 65, and the rates continue to increase with age. The increase in life expectancy will therefore place additional strains on the service, the consequences of which have been described in a slightly cynical but certainly challenging manner: '[T]he number of old fogies like me is mounting. When the baby boomers slide into decrepitude, they will be lucky to even get a bedpan.'[1]

Many years ago *The Times* invited readers to send in essays on the theme 'What is wrong with the world?' In response, GK Chesterton wrote:

'I am.'
Yours truly,
GK Chesterton

The same question is often asked of the health service and it may well be that we should adopt the position of Chesterton, and point the finger of blame at ourselves, asking whether, as members of the public, we have realistic aspirations and expectations of what the health service and the professionals, who provide care and treatment, can accomplish. Advancements in knowledge and changing practices have meant that diseases that for our parents' generation would have resulted in death or severe debilitation are now treatable and, in many cases, preventable. Despite these developments, utilisation rates for health services continue to increase based on perceptions that health care services can meet a greater proportion of our needs. In 1998 around 14% of people had consulted a GP in the previous 14 days, compared to around 11% in 1975.[2] The explanation for such a growth in utilisation can be partly attributed to the increase in the number of older people, but questions also have to be asked as to what motivates people to seek a consultation with a health care professional. For instance, recently a complaint was made against a consultant physician who diagnosed bronchitis rather than emphysema, which was what the patient 'wanted'!

As professionals, in adopting the position of Chesterton, it may be time to consider whether the critics of modern medicine are right when they say that medicine has outworn its welcome and its determination to produce perfect health.[1,3] It was Ivan Illich who argued that 'the major threat to health in the world is modern medicine'[3,4] and there have been calls from eminent professionals that his message, of over 30 years ago, receives the recognition it warrants.[5,6]

The WHO's definition of health – 'a state of complete physical, mental and social well-being, and not merely the absence of disease or infirmity'[7] – may have passed its sell by date.[1,8] For Illich, health is the capacity to cope with the human reality of death, pain and sickness, whereas modern medicine has sought to eradicate death, pain and sickness.[3,5] Illich portrays three levels of iatrogenesis:

(1) clinical iatrogenesis – the injury done to patients by ineffective, toxic and unsafe treatments, aspects of which have been highlighted in earlier chapters;

(2) social iatrogenesis – the results of the medicalisation of life, with more and more problems seen as amenable to medical intervention; and

(3) cultural iatrogenesis – the destruction of traditional ways of dealing with and making sense of death, pain and sickness.[3,4]

Others have also questioned the role of modern medicine.[1,9–11] For example, it has been claimed that:

> Health is not a 'state of complete physical, mental and social well-being', it is a capacity, despite the vicissitudes of life, to find 'a place in the sun' and a chance to add to the rich panoply of life. Not all our ills require expensive treatment: some do better without. By relinquishing our hypochrondiacal determination to find a cure (or a compensation)

for every ill, we might succeed in designing health care services that are accessible when we need them and sufficiently solvent to allow us to incorporate and make available some of the exciting medical innovations that will result from our knowledge of the human genome.[1]

On the other hand, there may be some encouraging signs – for example, the reflections of Lance Armstrong (six-time winner of one of the most gruelling and demanding of sporting events, the Tour de France cycle race) following testicular cancer are powerful and emotive, but also challenge those who follow the line of reasoning that all people have something wrong with them and that everyone and everything can be cured.[3,5]

> The experience of suffering is like the experience of exploring, of finding something unexpected and revelatory. When you find the outermost thresholds of pain, or fear, or uncertainty, what you experience afterwards is an expansive feeling, a widening of your capabilities .... Pain is good because it teaches your body and your soul to improve. It's almost as though your unconscious says, 'I'm going to remember this, remember how it hurt, and I'll increase my capacities so that the next time, it doesn't hurt as much'.[12]

The positive attitude displayed by Armstrong needs to be more evident in the demands that are placed on health care services, since the capacity of health care systems to actually deliver against ever-increasing demands on its resources is becoming more and more strained. The health care dilemma and attempts to address it have been a consistent theme throughout this book, but as the proportion of the population that reaches 'old age' increases, the pressures and the extent of the dilemma mount. 'We may choose to believe that health care is our right, but unless we make some changes in our health care delivery systems, health care will not be there when most of us would like it to be unless, of course, we are prepared to actually pay directly for it.'[1,13]

Health and its management is an area that cries out for a system based on *joined-up thinking* rather than one which is narrowly focused and driven by budgets. In recent times, the multiplicity of reforms and reorganisations, within the UK, have seen the NHS becoming fragmented, with the establishment of organisational and budgetary boundaries, resulting in many examples of service provision being driven by budgets, without due consideration for the impact of such decisions on the consequences for patients and health care provision in other areas.

Health care systems can be likened to the course of a river, from the relative simplicity of its structure and form at source to the complexity, magnitude and power at its confluence with the sea. Along its course the journey is influenced by many factors, while the river itself also has an effect on the communities and areas through which it flows. The same is true of health care systems. As patients enter the system and present with their health care problems, their interaction with health care professionals is relatively straightforward and simple to comprehend. However, the further they journey through the system, the degree of complexity intensifies, with many obstacles and problems to negotiate. As the patient reaches the hospital, he or she is subjected to an entirely different environment, just as the river is subjected to the tidal flows and other positive and negative effects as it joins the sea. What is also evident is that there is a direct correlation between the costs of dealing with health care problems and the location of the patient in the health care system – in simple terms, hospital costs are significantly greater than primary care costs, which means that it is much cheaper to 'fish patients out of the NHS river' nearer its source than when it enters the sea. To extend the analogy further, it is probably more efficient to prevent the patient from falling into the river in the first place.

Therefore, the adoption of a broader agenda in health policy would mean that one of the major objectives in decision-making would be to reduce the likelihood of acute episodes from becoming chronic. This would involve an investment of resources at early stages in the health care spectrum, dealing with problems at the outset, with the aim of removing people from the health care system rather than 'moving them on' to a more complex and expensive part of the system. More work is needed to develop a broader, strategic agenda in health care policy and decision-making and health economics can play an important role.

Health economics, as a discipline, has come a long way in a relatively short period of time. It probably took off in the 1970s, since when the subject and number of health economists have proliferated.[14] The growth in demand for health economic evaluations and the development of the pharmacoeconomic 'industry' for the purposes of pricing, reimbursement and formulary decision-making have burgeoned, but, as highlighted in Chapter 6, scepticism continues to exist. While there are grounds for suggesting that the levels of awareness and relevance of health economics are greater among clinicians and others in the health service at present,[14] the doubters still remain.[15–17]

Recent emphasis amongst health economists has tended to be on assessing the cost-effectiveness of treatments and particular health care interventions, rather than on preventive and public health schemes and programmes and considerations of the determinants of health. In Chapter 1, the issue was raised as to whether health care and the availability of health care facilities were the most important determinants in securing good health for society.[18] The question remains as to whether a greater focus on the determinants of health produces more health care benefits than investments in expensive treatments for a relatively small segment of the population.[11]

The initial Wanless Report in the UK highlighted the significance of chronic disease and the burden it was likely to pose for the NHS in the future – requiring an additional expenditure of £7.5 billion per year by 2010/11 across five chronic disease areas.[19] It has been estimated that a person with one chronic condition is likely to cost double that of a person without such a condition, but for a person with five or more chronic conditions, the differential is 14 times greater.[20] In the USA, such challenges have led to the development of chronic disease management models,[21,22] with an emphasis on preventive measures across different health care organisations. In the UK, although the NSFs seek to address the management of patients from a broad perspective, taking account of all stages in the disease process, there are large variations in hospitalisation rates associated with chronic diseases between different areas of the country.[23,24]

The management of chronic disease presents major challenges, but also provides opportunities. The challenges arise from the strain the disease imposes on patients and their families, and the pressures that the management of the disease exerts on the sustainability of formal heath systems and informal care support. These challenges are manifest in a variety of personal, economic and social effects, which impinge, to varying degrees, on a range of stakeholders. Concerted action that spans health care systems, other areas of government policy, non-governmental agencies, communities, patients and their families, with appropriate incentive schemes in place to address these challenges, is therefore required.

However, the management of chronic conditions also provides opportunities for coordinated approaches. While there are differences between diseases and their treatments, there are a number of common, related factors that can be an integral part of their management. For example, the role of poverty is a major causal ingredient in many chronic conditions, and policies designed to reduce and eliminate such a wide-ranging social problem will result in significant paybacks in many areas, including the reduction of chronic disease prevalence. Greater attention to the determinants of health and the development of a common set of protocols and guidelines, incorporated into a model of chronic disease management, could be an effective exploratory step in collectively addressing multiple comorbidities. What is needed is a move to establish frameworks and networks, which span organisational boundaries, based on partnership principles.[23,24] More work is needed to assess the positive effects of investing in relationships, within health care organisations and across organisational boundaries, to foster trust and collaboration across managerial and professional agendas[25] and to provide a service that seeks to prevent sickness and ill health, as well as treating problems once they arise. This was emphasised in the Acheson Report, which claimed that for too long the NHS had been viewed as a national sickness service rather than a national health service.[26]

The same principles apply to developing relationships and fostering trust and collaboration between health economists and other parties and bodies involved in the assessment of health care interventions, health care programmes and health care systems in general. While excessive expectations on the part of patients (and potential patients) as to what health care systems can actually accomplish, and unrealistic aspirations on the part of health care professionals as to what can be achieved in securing improvements in health may be partly responsible for the problems confronting the health service, and the same can be said for health economists.

The discipline of health economics 'has been distorted with too much effort being put into the broad advocacy of the techniques of economics evaluation and too little emphasis being placed both on methodological quality and development and on the broader application of the economics techniques to health policy'.[27] The propensity to bolt on economic evaluations to clinical studies and to model the economic impact of interventions following on from RCTs, without taking into consideration some of the broader issues and factors from the complex environment that impinge on the overall impact of treatments and therapies, has been very noticeable in the last few years, as the focus has switched more to the assessment and appraisal of health care technologies. As a result, it may be more appropriate to rename cost-effectiveness studies as cost-efficacy studies. And while valiant efforts are being made to deal with the effect of uncertainty so as to aid the decision-making process, the fact remains that the everyday world of health care is very different from the quasi-laboratory conditions under which clinical studies are undertaken, and, irrespective of the number of simulations of the available data, it is impossible to capture all possible scenarios and situations that might arise in the real world of clinical practice. Catastrophic adverse events, unforeseen circumstances that result in litigation and claims for compensation, changes in patients' preferences and perceptions, and other unintended consequences can all conspire to significantly affect the costs associated with a health care intervention, which was considered cost-effective at initial assessment. Similarly, the actual outcomes resulting from such interventions over a period of time, way in excess of the duration of any clinical study programme, cannot be confined to a single measure that encapsulates the effect on a single patient.

That is not to say that health economics has no relevance. Indeed, it has been argued that when resources are not used efficiently, unnecessary suffering and death result.[28] However, the problem with many health care systems is that they are fragmented and narrowly focused, with excessive significance attached to financial budgets, and insufficient attention paid to the wider picture and societal agenda, which has resulted in a very narrow perspective when assessing efficiency issues. Furthermore, there are grounds for believing that inequalities and inequities in health care, especially in terms of health status, are at best static and in all probability increasing.[29] Health economists have also fallen into the trap of being narrowly focused with regard to efficiency issues and have failed to grasp the bigger picture. Therefore, it is perhaps time to change the emphasis from the economics of health care to exploring the economics of health.[18] What has been advocated is that a broader perspective and set of approaches be employed,[30,31] whereby the economic framework would enable decision-makers (on behalf of society) to impute their own values to the profile of costs and consequences, which could differ according to local context, and where decision-makers would be able to clearly identify what is included and what is omitted.[31]

Health policy issues will always be high on political agendas and demands on health care resources will always outstrip the available supply. Techno-logical advancements, developments in medical science and increasing ex-pectations of communities as to what is available from health care providers continue to focus attention on the health care dilemma, which means that choices will always have to be made regarding the level of resources allocated to health care and, within health care, as to which areas receive a greater share and which receive less. In making such choices an explicit set of priorities needs to be established and attitudes changed. For example, the following argument states:

> A health care policy which embraces, through additional NHS re-sources, workplace health promotion, assistance to stop people smoking and encourages them to adopt healthier lifestyles would be welcome, explicitly recognising the positive relationship between health and work.... A healthier and wealthier workforce now will result in health-ier and wealthier pensioners in the future. Significant proportions of economically inactive individuals today will mean that as people move towards old age their need for health and social care services will increase. The current pressures on overstretched public services will continue to dominate media attention and government think tanks until governments commit themselves to joined-up policy making both on paper and in practice.... Moving money around the NHS will not deliver. We need to *work* our way today to ensure a healthier Wales in the future.[30]

Therefore, health economics has a contribution to make and it is unlikely that there will be many dissenting voices to the hope that health economics can be a resource that health care decision-makers can utilise to the benefit of patient care.[14] The evidence base for the effectiveness of health care interventions and programmes is continuously being developed. The recog-nition of the need to generate evidence relating to resource utilisation and the most beneficial utilisation of available resources is encouraging.

However, the existence of ineffectiveness and inefficiencies in service pro-vision has to be addressed. The development of evidence-based practice, a recognition that resources are finite and choices have to be made, and an awareness of the need for fairness in resource allocation and service provision are major steps along the road to answering the question of how much additional resources should be put into health care in general. What is left is the will to move along the road of change and make things happen.

References

1 Mallenson A. *Whiplash and other useful illnesses.* Montreal: McGill-Queen's University Press, 2002.

2 Yuen P. *Compendium of health statistics.* London: Office of Health Economics, 2000: Table 1.23.

3 Illich I. *Medical nemesis: the expropriation of health.* London: Calder and Boyars, 1975.

4 Illich I. Medical nemesis (reprint). *J Epidemiol Commun Health* 2003; 57: 919–22.

5 Smith R, Illich I. Limits to medicine. Medical nemesis: the expropriation of health. *J Epidemiol Commun Health* 2003; 57: 928.

6 Edwards RHT. Nemesis, Sisyphus, and a contribution from the medical humanities to health research. *J Epidemiol Commun Health* 2003; 57: 926–27.

7 World Health Organisation. *Official Records*, No. 2. Geneva: WHO, 1948.

8 Mooney G. *Economics, medicine and health care.* London: Harvester Wheatsheaf, 1992.

9 McKeown T. A historical appraisal of the medical task, in McLachlan, McKeown T (eds). *Medical history and medical care.* London: Nuffield Provincial Hospitals Trust, 1971.

10 McKeown T. *Medicine and modern society.* London: Allen and Unwin, 1965.

11 Evans RG, Stoddart GL. Producing health, consuming health care in Evans RG, Barer ML, Marmor TRE (eds). *Why are some people healthy and others are not? The determinants of health of populations.* New York: Aldine de Gruyter, 1994.

12 Armstrong L, Jenkins S. *Every second counts.* London: Yellow Jersey Press, 2003.

13 The Economist. A new prescription. *The Economist* 2000; 354: 29.

14 McCrone P. *Understanding health economics: a guide for health care decision makers.* London: Kogan Page, 1998.

15 Kernick DP. The impact of health economics on healthcare delivery: a primary care perspective. *Pharmacoeconomics* 2000; 18: 311–15.

16 Kernick D. Health economics: an evolving paradigm but sailing in the wrong direction? A view from the front line. *Health Econ* 2002; 11: 87–88.

17 Kernick DP. Has health economics lost its way? *BMJ* 1998; 317: 197–99.

18 Edwards RT. Paradigms and research programmes: is it time to move from health care economics to health economics. *Health Econ* 2001; 10: 635–49.

19 Wanless D. *Securing our future health: taking a long-term view.* London: HM Treasury, 2002. *http://www.hm-treasury.gov.uk/consultations_and_legislation/wanless/consult_wanless_index.cfm* (accessed 12 March 2004)

20 Partnership for Solutions, Johns Hopkins University, for The Robert Wood Johnson Foundation. *Chronic conditions: making the case for ongoing care.* Baltimore: Johns Hopkins University, 2002. ISBN 0–9727261-0-1. *http://www.partnershipforsolutions.org/DMS/files/chronicbook2002.pdf* (accessed 12 March 2004)

21 Wagner EH. Chronic disease management: what will it take to improve care for chronic illness? *Effective Clin Pract* 1998; 1: 2–4.

22 Bodenheimer T, Wagner EH, Grumbach K. Improving primary care for patients with chronic illness. *JAMA* 2002; 288: 1775–79.

23 Dixon J, Lewis R, Rosen R *et al. Managing chronic disease: what can we learn from the US experience?* London: Kings Fund, 2004.

24 Lewis R, Dixon J. Rethinking management of chronic diseases. *BMJ* 2004; 328: 220–22.

25 Mitton C, Donaldson C. *Priority setting tool kit: a guide to the use of economics in healthcare decision making.* London: BMJ Books, 2004.

26 Independent inquiry into inequalities in health. *The Acheson Report.* London: HMSO, 1998.

27 Maynard A, Sheldon TA. Health economics: has it fulfilled its potential? in Maynard A, Chalmers I (eds). *Non-random reflections on health services research: on the 25th anniversary of Archie Cochrane's 'Effectiveness and Efficiency'.* London: BMJ Books, 1997.

28 Williams A. Ethics, clinical freedom and the doctors' role, in Culyer AJ, Maynard A, Pornett J. (eds). *Competition in health care: reforming the NHS.* Basingstoke: Macmillan, 1990.

29 Evans R. *Interpreting and addressing inequalities in health: from Black to Acheson to Blair to . . . ?* London: Office of Health Economics, 2002.

30 Phillips CJ, Edwards RT. The economics of health in Wales. *Welsh Econ Rev* 2003; 14: 26–30.

31 Coast J. Is economic evaluation in touch with society's health values? *BMJ* 2004; 329: 1233–36.

Index